seventh edition

Anybody's
Guide to
TOTAL
FITNESS

Len Kravitz

University of New Mexico

KENDALL/HUNT PUBLISHING COMPANY
4050 Westmark Drive   Dubuque, Iowa 52002

W9-AYZ-525

Chairman and Chief Executive Officer   Mark C. Falb
Vice President, Director of National Book Program   Alfred C. Grisanti
Editorial Development Supervisor   Georgia Botsford
Developmental Editor   Tina Bower
Prepress Project Coordinator   Sheri Hosek
Prepress Editor   Charmayne McMurray
Design Manager   Jodi Splinter
Senior Vice President, College Division   Thomas W. Gantz
Vice President and National Field Manager   Brian Johnson
Managing Editor, College Field   Paul Carty
Associate Editor, College Field   Jay Hays

Illustrations by Jill Pankey

Cover photos (from top to bottom) courtesy of:
1 and 7 © 2003 Corbis
2, 4, 5, 6, 8, 9, and 10 © 2003 PhotoDisc, Inc.
3 and 11 © 2003 Digital Stock
Main image © 2003 PhotoDisc, Inc.

Copyright © 1986, 1989, 1992, 1995, 1998, 2000 by Len Kravitz
Copyright © 2003 by Kendall/Hunt Publishing Company

ISBN 0-7872-9878-1

All rights reserved. No part of this publication may be reproduced,
stored in a retrieval system, or transmitted, in any form or by any
means, electronic, mechanical, photocopying, recording, or otherwise,
without the prior written permission of the copyright owner.

Printed in the United States of America
10 9 8 7 6 5 4 3 2 1

Dedicated with love to my mom,
who always believed in me

CONTENTS

SECTION 5
Contemporary Health Issues   101

SECTION 6
Fitness Facts and Fiction   127

ACKNOWLEDGMENTS

I would like to express my deep appreciation and gratitude to my original editorial advisory board of Dr. Carol L. Christensen, Dr. Craig J. Cisar, Dr. Gail G. Evans, Dr. Susan Kutner, Lori Leeds, R.P.T., Dr. Thomas A. MacLean, Dr. Susan Pate, Dr. Robert Pearl, Dr. Jay D. Pruzansky, Dr. Norman T. Reynolds, Richard V. Schroeder, M.S., and Dr. Phillip A. Sienna. Their advice, expertise, and thoughtful review of this book were invaluable.

I sincerely thank the following people who have made generous contributions to this project and deserve special acknowledgement: Emmanuel Athans, Molly Burke, Mert and Tanya Carpenter, Kim Drummond, Janice Earle, Carrie Ekins, Eric Finch, Dixie Fisher, Sue Forster-Cox, Glenda Gilliam, Marla Graves, Jerry Gonsalves, Jean Harding, Louise Herndon, Michael Le Doux, Shirley H. M. Reekie, Pauline Reimer, Joe Samuels, Wendy Russum, Dolores Sargent, Amy Scofield, Carol Stewart, Ph.D., Debbie Sporleder, Carol Sullivan, Pamela Staver, and Teri Wexted.

I would also like to thank the following special people who have been a source of inspiration and have guided me in countless ways: Covert Bailey, Dr. Barton Byers, Dr. Laurence Berkowitz, Ed and Shirley Burke, Don Callahan, Roy Cerrito, Retta Chavkin, Dr. Barbara Conry, Yvonne Cotton, Peter and Kathie Davis, Anita Del Grande, Jerry Dollard, Dr. Jacqueline Douglass, Ronda Gates, Dr. Telemachos A. Greanias, Dr. William F. Gustafson, C. Lansing Hays, Ellen Herbst, Dr. Vivian H. Heyward, Dr. Clair W. Jennett, DeAun Kizer, Bob Kravitz, Joyce Malone, Frank Napier, Dr. Bruce Ogilvie, Lawrence R. Petulla, Doug Sporleder, Marty Urand, and Neil Wiley.

For their enthusiastic support, I am grateful to my friends at the Los Gatos Athletic Club, the faculty and staff of Human Performance at San Jose State University, and everyone at Aerobics Plus.

I am also deeply indebted to my friend Chuck Drummond for providing such wise counsel and friendship.

To Dr. Susan Pate, my original editor and lifetime friend, I thank you in a thousand different ways.

To Jill Pankey, my illustrator, I thank you for your artistic imagination and for the many hours of hard work you devoted to this book to make it come to life.

WELCOME TO A HEALTHY WAY OF LIFE

Living and enjoying life to its fullest is a wonderful goal. And you can have it! Fitness is a way of life that allows you to function and perform at your best. It's a harmonic balance of prescribed exercise, healthy eating habits, preventative health care, effective stress management, and a common-sense lifestyle. Your level of fitness helps determine the quality of your life. You are in control of how you look, feel, and live.

The following information is based on sound physiological principles and research. With a minimal investment of your time, you can follow these concepts and create a fitness plan that will help you obtain the most from your life.

I have presented a specific aerobics program for you. You may wish to supplement it with a running, swimming, or cycling program of your own.

Be patient, use your knowledge, set your goals, listen to your body, and commit yourself to a healthy way of life.

ABOUT THE AUTHOR

Len Kravitz, Ph.D., is the coordinator of Exercise Science at the University of New Mexico where he received his doctorate with an emphasis in Health Promotion and Exercise Science. Dr. Kravitz was voted the 1999 International Presenter of the Year by the Canadian Professional Fitness Association and was the first person to win the IDEA Fitness Instructor of the Year award (1997). Len has authored more than 100 articles on health and fitness for several national publications and has been featured on *CNN News, Dateline* and *CBS This Morning.*

Dr. Kravitz is a versatile movement specialist with a broad range of skills, which include competitive gymnastics at the national and international levels and professional theater/mime performances on stage and video. He is the creator of *Anybody's Workout, Anybody's 3-in-1 Workout, Anybody's Step Workout,* and the *SuperAbs* exercise videos, which have been featured in national magazines and TV shows. Len's innovative technique and teaching style have made him a sought-after lecturer for fitness professionals around the United States, Canada, Europe, Taiwan, and Japan.

Section 1

STARTING OUT

What Exercise Will Do for You

Benefits of a well-balanced health and fitness program are:

- ❑ A healthy appearance

- ❑ Good posture and alignment

- ❑ Fluid, easy movement

- ❑ Stronger joints and firmer muscles

- ❑ Lowered risk for low-back pain

- ❑ A decreased susceptibility to injury

- ❑ Fewer aches and pains

- ❑ A more efficient circulatory and respiratory system

- ❑ Lowered risk of cardiovascular disease and stroke

- ❑ Improved blood cholesterol levels

- ❑ Better control of blood pressure

- ❑ Increased life expectancy

- ❑ A decrease in body fat and/or body weight

- ❑ Controlled appetite

- ❑ Better digestion

- ❑ Improved mental awareness, self-esteem, and self-confidence

- ❑ Improved ability to relax

- ❑ Better handling of stress

- ❑ Help in preventing and coping with depression

- ❑ More restful sleep

- ❑ Increased job productivity

- ❑ More energy and vitality

- ❑ AN INCREASED ABILITY TO ENJOY LIFE

Stickin' to It!

Tips for Exercise Success

These tips will steer you toward success in exercise.

1. **Write out a health and fitness evaluation list**—what you do right (don't smoke, good eating habits, no substance abuse, etc.) and what you need to correct (lack of regular exercise, posture, high emotional stress, etc.). Then figure out what you can do to shift more entries to the "right" side.

2. **Set realistic long- and short-term goals.** Make sure you break them down into manageable steps. Write this out like a personal contract, including objectives of your health and fitness action plan and the date you plan to start specific activities. Solicit the support of someone close to you. Keep track of your progress, revising your fitness plan if needed, and reward yourself as goals are achieved (a show, a new outfit, a book, etc.).

3. **Find a workout companion** with a fitness level and goals similar to yours. Pick some exercise activities or classes that you both enjoy, and commit to participating in them. Talk to other individuals who have reached goals similar to yours. Find out what strategies helped them keep on track.

> ### Did You Know?
> More than half of the people who start an exercise program drop out after six months.

4. **Schedule your exercise three to five days per week.** Choose a "special" time of day, and be selfish about preserving that time for your body and general well-being.

5. **Listen to your body and progress slowly in the beginning.** Most injuries in fitness come from doing too much, too soon, too fast, and too hard.

6. **Don't let early awkwardness or uneven skill development get you down.** It happens to everyone). And try not to compare yourself to others.

7. **Wear comfortable exercise clothing and proper shoes.** Your clothing should permit you to move freely and allow your body to cool itself. Do not wear fabrics that hinder evaporation.

8. **Plan your exercise** at least two hours after or at least an hour before a big meal.

9. **Be patient;** exercise has many immediate and delayed benefits. Your time will come! Don't get angry at yourself if you miss a workout or slip on a health goal. Try to focus on what caused the lapse and how you may better deal with it in the future. Most importantly, stay positive and believe in yourself. You are in control.

10. **Be aware of the signs of overexertion:** breathlessness, dizziness, tightness or pain in the chest, loss of muscle control, and nausea. If you experience any of these signs, stop immediately. See your physician to determine the cause. Also, don't exercise if you are sick.

Five Key Components of Fitness

Your body is a complex mechanism designed for action. Being physically fit means that the heart, blood vessels, lungs, and muscles function at optimal efficiency. Following are five key components of health-related physical fitness with which you need to be concerned.

1. **Cardiorespiratory Endurance/Aerobic Conditioning** is the ability of the body's heart, lungs, blood vessels, and major muscle groups to persist in continuous rhythmic exercise such as brisk walking, jogging, swimming, aerobics, rowing, cycling, step training, skating, and cross-country skiing. Regular aerobic conditioning may prevent or reduce the likelihood of cardiovascular disease. Cardiorespiratory endurance is the most important component of health-related fitness.

2. **Muscular Strength** is the ability of the muscles to exert maximal or near maximal force against resistance. Stronger muscles protect the joints that they surround and reduce the incidence of injury from physical activity.

   An increase in muscle mass will also boost the body's metabolism.

3. **Muscular Endurance** is the ability of skeletal muscle to exert force (not necessarily maximal) over an extended period of time. Strength, skill, performance, speed of movement, and power are closely associated with this component. Muscular endurance helps to prevent injuries and improve posture.

4. **Flexibility** is the range of motion of the muscles and joints of the body. It has to do with your skeletal muscles' natural and conditioned ability to extend beyond their normal resting length. Increased flexibility will enhance performance and reduce the incidence of injury.

5. **Body Composition** is the relationship of percentage of body fat to lean body weight (muscle, bone, water, vital organs). Being overfat, which usually starts in childhood, has a limiting effect on the other components of fitness. High body fat is associated with a number of health problems including heart disease, high blood pressure, stroke, diabetes, cancer and back pain.

Energy for Exercise

To exercise and do work for daily activities, your body uses a chemical called ATP (adenosine triphosphate) like a car uses gasoline. ATP is produced by metabolizing the foods you eat, particularly carbohydrates and fats. Depending on the intensity and duration of the activity, you produce ATP through aerobic and/or anaerobic metabolism.

Aerobic (with oxygen) metabolism is the most efficient and main energy production system. This metabolic pathway cannot work unless there is sufficient oxygen available in the tissues during exercise. Prolonged vigorous activity over five minutes activates your aerobic metabolism; however, at least 20 minutes of this kind of activity is recommended to enhance your aerobic capacity.

Anaerobic (without oxygen) metabolism is used for situations requiring quick bursts of energy, such as lifting weights, running short races, jumping, and throwing. Although it is less efficient than the aerobic system, it can quickly generate the ATP needed at the muscle site. Anaerobic metabolism may be called on during aerobic conditioning if your intensity increases beyond the ability of your system to deliver oxygen (such as finishing a long run with a sprint or a section of high kicks during an aerobic program).

On Your Mark, Get Set . . . Wait!

It is always a good idea to undergo a medical examination before embarking on a strenuous program of exercise.

With your physician, write up a personal medical profile including a history of high blood pressure, chest pain, heart arrhythmia, or shortness of breath. Determine your coronary heart disease risk. Here's a list of heart disease risk factors and what you can do about them.

Risk Factor	Criteria
Positive Risk Factors	
Family history	Myocardial infarction or sudden death before 55 years of age in father or other male first-degree relative (i.e., brother or son) or before 65 years of age in mother or female first-degree relative (i.e., sister or daughter)
Cigarette smoking	Current cigarette smoker or those who quit within previous 6 months
High blood pressure	Systolic blood pressure ≥ 140 mmHg or diastolic ≥ 90 mmHg (confirmed on two separate occasions) or taking antihypertensive medication
Hypercholesterolemia	Total serum cholesterol > 200 mg/dL, or high-density lipoprotein cholesterol < 35 mg/dL, or on lipid-lowering medication. If LDL-C is available, use > 130 mg/dL rather than total cholesterol.
Impaired fasting glucose	Fasting blood glucose of ≥ 110 mg/dL (confirmed on at least two separate occasions)
Obesity	Body Mass Index of ≥ 30 kg/m² or waist girth 100 cm
Sedentary lifestyle	Persons not participating in a regular exercise program or meeting the minimal physical activity recommendations from the U.S. Surgeon General's report (accumulating 30 minutes or more of moderate intensity physical activity on most days of the week)
Negative Risk Factor	
High serum HDL-C	> 60 ml/dL of high density lipoprotein cholesterol

Note: Positive risk factors PROMOTE disease whereas negative risk factors NEGATE disease

How Fit Are You?

Here are some simple self-assessment tests to help determine or monitor your level of fitness. Periodically retest yourself to monitor your progress. (Stop) if you feel any nausea, discomfort, dizziness, or breathlessness. Perform the test on another day.

Aerobic Efficiency

Step Test

1. Select a bench, stool, or chair that is 12 inches high.

2. You will step up and down in an up, up, down, down brisk cadence.

3. Find a song that has a moderate tempo of about 96 beats per minute (16 beats in 10 seconds) to guide your cadence.

4. Rehearse stepping with the music to become familiar with the pattern.

5. Practice finding your pulse on your wrist (on the inner edge of the wrist below the base of the thumb) or at your neck (below the ear along the jaw).

6. Now, perform the stepping for three continuous minutes. On completion of the time, immediately count your pulse for 10 seconds.

7. Record score and rating in the *Student Profile Guide* on page 11.

Step Test Rating (Counting pulse for 10 seconds)			
Level	**Women**	**Men**	
Excellent	16 or less	17 or less	Congratulations!
Good	17–18	18–20	Keep it up!
Fair	19–22	21–23	Begin or progress in an aerobic program.
Poor	23 or more	24 or more	Start with a moderate to easy aerobic program.

(Test based on the Harvard Step Test.)

1.5-Mile Run Test

1. Establish a distance of 1.5 miles. This is six laps around most school tracks (which are usually one-quarter mile).

2. Use a stopwatch to time yourself.

3. Warm up with some easy jogging and gentle stretching before you start.

4. Cover the distance as fast as you can (running/walking). Cool down gradually at the conclusion with brisk walking for several minutes.

5. Record score and rating in the *Student Profile Guide* on page 12.

Rating the 1.5-Mile Run Time (Minutes)

Fitness Category		13–19	20–29	30–39	40–49	50–59	60+
				Age (years)			
I. Very poor	(men)	>15:31*	>16:01	>16:31	>17:31	>19:01	>20:01
	(women)	>18:31	>19:01	>19:31	>20:01	>20:31	>21:01
II. Poor	(men)	12:11–15:30	14:01–16:00	14:44–16:30	15:36–17:30	17:01–19:00	19:01–20:00
	(women)	16:55–18:30	18:31–19:00	19:01–19:30	19:01–20:00	20:01–20:30	21:00–21:31
III. Fair	(men)	10:49–12:10	12:01–14:00	12:31–14:45	13:01–15:35	14:31–17:00	16:16–19:00
	(women)	14:31–16:54	15:55–18:30	16:31–19:00	17:31–19:30	19:01–20:00	19:31–20:30
IV. Good	(men)	9:41–10:48	10:46–12:00	11:01–12:30	11:31–13:00	12:31–14:30	14:00–16:15
	(women)	12:30–14:30	13:31–15:54	14:31–16:30	15:56–17:30	16:31–19:00	17:31–19:30
V. Excellent	(men)	8:37–9:40	9:45–10:45	10:00–11:00	10:30–11:30	11:00–12:30	11:15–13:59
	(women)	11:50–12:29	12:30–13:30	13:00–14:30	13:45–15:55	14:30–16:30	16:30–17:30
VI. Superior	(men)	<8:37	<9:45	<10:00	<10:30	<11:00	<11:15
	(women)	<11:50	<12:30	<13:00	<13:45	<14:30	<16:30

< Means "less than"; > means "more than."

"1.5 mile run tests," from *The Aerobics Program for Total Well Being* by Kenneth H. Cooper M.D., M.P.H, Copyright © 1982 by Kenneth H. Cooper. Used by permission of Bantam Books, a division of Bantam Doubleday Dell Publishing Group, Inc.

Rockport Fitness Walking Test

The Rockport Walking Institute has developed a walking test to assess cardiorespiratory fitness for men and women ages 20–69.

1. Find a 1-mile course that is flat, uninterrupted, and correctly measured. A quarter-mile track is preferable.

2. Walk 1 mile as quickly and comfortably as possible.

3. Immediately take a heart rate by counting your pulse for 15 seconds and multiplying that number by four (to get your heart for one minute).

4. Record your score and rating in the *Student Profile Guide* on page 13.

Use the Rockport relative fitness charts on pages 12 and 13 to classify your cardiorespiratory fitness. The walking time and corresponding postexercise heart rate are located on the appropriate chart for your age and gender. These charts are based on body weights of 125 lb. for women and 170 lb. for men. If you weigh substantially more than this value, your cardiorespiratory fitness level will be overestimated.

Rating the Rockport Fitness Walking Test

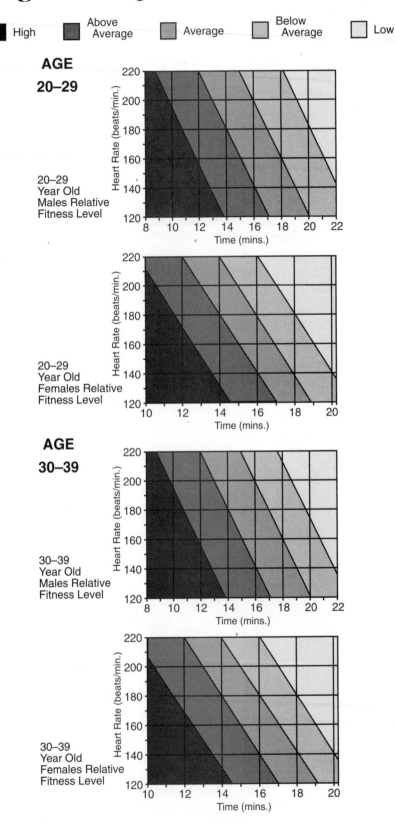

Legend: High | Above Average | Average | Below Average | Low

AGE 20–29

20–29 Year Old Males Relative Fitness Level

20–29 Year Old Females Relative Fitness Level

AGE 30–39

30–39 Year Old Males Relative Fitness Level

30–39 Year Old Females Relative Fitness Level

Rating the Rockport Fitness Walking Test

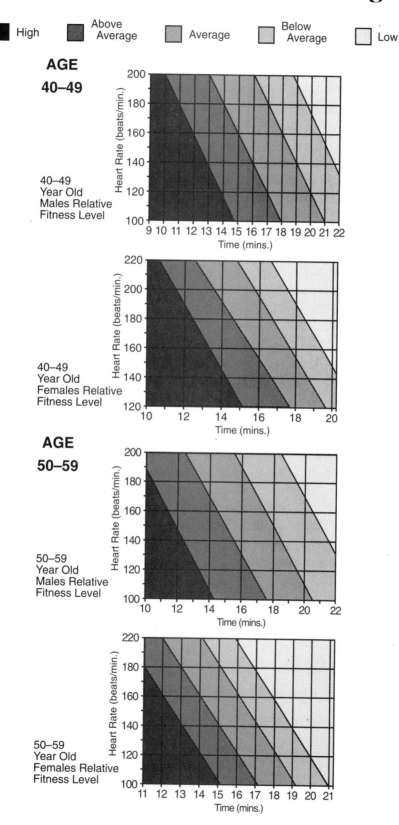

■ High   ■ Above Average   ▦ Average   ▦ Below Average   □ Low

AGE 40–49

40–49 Year Old Males Relative Fitness Level

40–49 Year Old Females Relative Fitness Level

AGE 50–59

50–59 Year Old Males Relative Fitness Level

50–59 Year Old Females Relative Fitness Level

Muscular Strength and Endurance

Abdominal Strength and Endurance Test

1. Lie on your back with your hands either supporting your head or across you chest.

2. Keep your legs bent at the knees, with the feet flat on the floor about 6 to 10 inches from your buttocks.

3. To perform the "crunch," curl your trunk so that your shoulder blades come off the floor. (Your lower back stays on the floor.) Keep it smooth.

4. To take the test, count the number of "crunches" you can do for one minute.

5. Record results and rating in the *Student Profile Guide* on page 14.

Rating for Abdominal Strength and Endurance Test	
Category	**Results**
Excellent	60 crunches or more
Very Good	50 to 59 crunches
Good	42 to 49 crunches
Fair	34 to 41 crunches
Poor	Less than 34 crunches

Upper Torso Strength and Endurance Test

The push-up may be completed in the standard style (with the body straight and supported by the hands and feet) or the modified style (with the knees on the ground).

1. Lower the chest so it almost makes contact with the floor and then straighten the arms.

2. To take the test, count the total number of push-ups completed in one minute.

3. Start with the modified push-up. Once you have reached the "excellent level" with the modified push-up, proceed to the standard push-up.

4. Record results and rating in the *Student Profile Guide* on page 15.

Rating for Upper Torso Strength and Endurance Test		
	Modified Push-ups[1]	**Standard Push-ups[2]**
Excellent	31 push-ups or more	41 push-ups or more
Very Good	21 to 30 push-ups	30 to 40 push-ups
Good	18 to 20 push-ups	24 to 29 push-ups
Fair	13 to 17 push-ups	18 to 23 push-ups
Poor	Less than 7 push-ups	Less than 12 push-ups

[1] Norms for women only. Adapted from Heyward, V. H. (2002). Advanced fitness assessment and exercise prescription. Human Kinetics, 2002.

[2] Norms for men only. Adapted from Heyward, V. H. (2002). Advanced fitness assessment and exercise prescription. Human Kinetics, 2002.

Flexibility

Sit-and-Reach Test

Flexibility is specific. This means that the degree of flexibility in one joint will not necessarily be the same in other joints of the body. Because a lack of flexibility in the lower back, back of the legs, and hips is a contributing cause for 80 percent of lower-back problems of our population, this flexibility test was chosen.

1. Sit with your legs extended in front of you. Keep your feel perpendicular to the floor. Place a ruler along your legs on the floor.

2. Slowly stretch forward, reaching toward (or past) your toes and hold. (Do not bounce!) Keep your legs straight but not locked.

3. It is best to do this several times for practice, gently stretching further toward your point of limitation.

4. Record results and rating in the *Student Profile Guide* on page 16.

Ratings for the Sit-and-Reach Test	
Category	**Results**
Excellent	7 inches or more past the toes
Very Good	4 to 7 inches past the toes
Good	1 to 4 inches past the toes
Fair	2 inches from in front of the toes to 1 inch past
Poor	More than 2 inches in front of the toes

A limitation of this sit-and-reach test is that it does not differentiate between a person with short arms and/or long legs and someone with long arms and/or short legs. However, this test is very applicable to monitor flexibility changes over time.

Body Composition

Pinch Test for Body Fat

The pinch test is a quick check for body composition. (You can always count on the mirror to tell you a lot, too!)

1. With your thumb and forefinger, pinch the skin and fat at the waist just above the hips. (Be sure not to pinch any muscle. Pull the skinfold away from your body.)

2. With a ruler measure the width of the pinch.

3. Record results and rating in the *Student Profile Guide* on page 17.

Ratings for Pinch Test		
Level	Men	Women
Good to Excellent	1/2 inch or less	1 inch or less
Fair to Good	1 inch to 1/2	1 1/2 inch to 1 inch
Poor	Over 1 inch	Over 1 1/2 inch

Refer to Skinfold Caliper Measurement for a more accurate estimate of body composition.

Skinfold Caliper Measurement

Approximately one-third of the fat in the body is located just under the skin and is closely correlated to total body fat. Researchers have demonstrated that this skinfold fat is distributed differently in men and women and, for that reason, skinfold measurements are taken at different body locations. Skinfolds should not be taken immediately after exercise, because the shift of body fluids will increase the skinfold size.

There are several practical and inexpensive skinfold calipers available for body composition analysis. To take a skinfold measurement,

1. Grasp the anatomical site with the thumb and index finger.

2. Lift the skinfold away from the site to make sure no muscle is caught in the fold.

3. Place the caliper one-half inch below the thumb and index finger.

4. Allow the caliper to stabilize for a few seconds before reading. Take at least three measurements, and record the average.

5. Total the average of your skinfolds.

6. Determine your percentage of body fat by placing a straightedge from your age to the sum of the three skinfolds on the nomogram. The recommended percentage of body fat is 16 to 25 percent for a woman and 12 to 18 percent for a man. There is an error factor of plus or minus 3 to 5 percent with skinfold body composition assessment.

7. Record the results and rating in the *Student Profile Guide* on page 18.

Skinfolds are conventionally taken on the right side of the body. Here is how to find the anatomical skinfold sites:

- ❑ **Chest**—the fold over the side border of the pectoralis major

- ❑ **Abdomen**—vertical fold adjacent to the umbilicus

- ❑ **Thigh**—vertical fold on the front part of the thigh midway between the hip and knee joint

- ❑ **Triceps**—vertical fold on the back of the arm midway between the shoulder and elbow (arm held straight and relaxed)

- ❑ **Suprailium**—diagonal fold above the crest of the ilium

Anatomical Skinfold Sites

Skinfold Nomogram

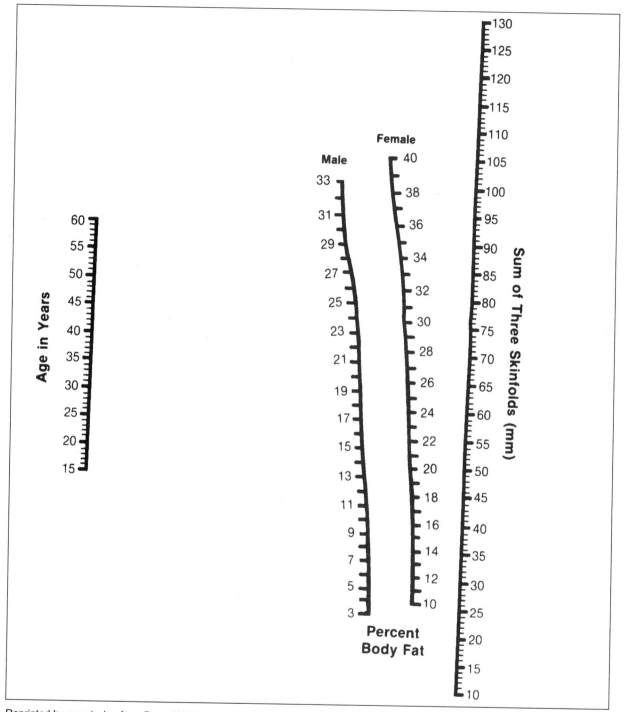

Reprinted by permission from Baun, W. B. Baun, M. R. A Nomogram for the Estimate of Percent Body Fat from Generalized Equations. *Research Quarterly for Exercise and Sport,* 52 (1981), 380–384.

The "S.P.O.R.T." Principle

Fitness conditioning involves the "S.P.O.R.T." principle: Specificity, Progression, Overload, Reversibility, and Training Effect.

Specificity: Specificity takes the guesswork out of training. Your body will adapt to the specific type of training you choose. If you want to run marathons, you've got to train long distances. If you wish to build muscles, you must do intense weight training. Identify your goals and get started.

Progression: Challenge your body's abilities gradually and regularly. Let your body adapt to its new capability, and then you can progress some more. (Injuries happen from trying to do too much, too soon, too hard, and too fast.)

Overload: You "overload" by increasing the intensity, duration, or frequency of your established level of exercise. For instance, you may do aerobics longer, more times a week, or at a more intense level. When your exercise program becomes easier and somewhat routine, it is often a good time to overload. Overload your exercise program in increments of about 5 percent of your present ability.

Reversibility: You can't store the benefits of exercise. If you stop exercising there will be a marked decrease in skill, endurance, and strength from your previous level. So keep it up!

Training Effect: As you specifically train for a certain activity, you gradually and progressively overload your body's ability. The resulting increase in muscular and cardiorespiratory conditioning is the training effect.

Your final phase is to **MAINTAIN** this newly acquired level of health throughout your lifetime. You can do it!

The Formula for Aerobic Fitness

To benefit from a sound cardiorespiratory program, follow the "F.I.T." formula. "F.I.T." stands for Frequency, Intensity, and Time.

Frequency: For optimal results, perform your aerobic activity three to five times a week (preferably every other day). If you choose to exercise more, make sure you rest at least one day each week to prevent any injuries from overuse!

Intensity: Your intensity should be 50 percent to 85 percent of your personalized training zone. For beginners in good health, 60 percent to 70 percent of your training zone is encouraged.

Time: The time or duration should gradually build up to between 20 and 60 minutes.

> **Did You Know?**
>
> Only 15 percent of all adults exercise regularly enough to promote health-related fitness.

Heart Rate Monitoring

Monitoring your heart rate is a very simple, practical, and safe way to understand your exertion during aerobics. You will improve your cardiorespiratory system if you train at 60 percent to 85 percent of your personalized target zone. To estimate your target zone, you must first calculate your maximum heart rate and your resting heart rate. Your maximum heart rate (the fastest

Personalized Target Zone		
Constant	220	
Your age	− 30	
Subtract age from constant; this equals estimated maximum heart rate	= 190	
Your resting heart rate	− 72	
Subtract resting heart rate from estimated maximum heart rate	= 118	
Multiply by	60%	85%
Equals	71	100
Add resting heart rate	+ 72	+ 72
Equals exercise heart rate	143	172
	Target Zone	

Personalized Target Zone		
Constant	220	
Your age		
Subtract age from constant; this equals estimated maximum heart rate		
Your resting heart rate		
Subtract resting heart rate from estimated maximum heart rate		
Multiply by	60%	85%
Equals		
Add resting heart rate		
Equals exercise heart rate		
	Target Zone	

your heart will beat) can be estimated by subtracting your age from 220. Resting heart rate is defined as the average heart rate (per minute) prior to initiating any physical activity. It is often measured in the morning, after waking up, and prior to physical activity. Here's how a 30-year-old individual with a resting heart rate of 72 would estimate her personalized target zone.

1. Find your pulse with your index and middle fingers pressed gently on your wrist (on the inner edge of the wrist below the base of the thumb) or neck (below the ear along the jaw) and count for 10 seconds.

2. Multiply by 6 to find the beats per minute. Pulse monitoring at the wrist is recommended because you can inadvertently press too hard on the neck and cause a slowing of the heart rate.

3. Monitor your heart rate before, after three to five minutes of aerobic exercise, and on completion of an aerobic section. Keep moving while you take your exercise pulse.

Some students find it easy to calculate their personalized target zone for a 10-second count. To do this, divide your exercise heart rate by 6. For instance, if your personalized target zone is 150 beats per minute to 180 beats per minute, your 10-second count would be determined as follows: 150/6 = 25; 180/6 = 30. So, if you do a 10-second pulse check while exercising, your heart rate should be between 25 and 30.

Perceived Exertion

You can also monitor exercise intensity through the use of perceived exertion. With perceived exertion, you interpret various body sensations such as heart rate, muscle and joint sensations, breathing intensity, and body temperature, and subjectively estimate your exercise intensity. A model that corresponds exercise heart rate with perceived exertion has been developed by Gunnar Borg, a Swedish physiologist. Notice that by adding a "0" to the numbers of the perceived exertion scale, it correlates to your exercise heart rate intensity. This is a great way to learn to listen to your body and compare your results to your counted heart rate. An easy way to know if you are within your ideal aerobic exercise intensity is to perceptually monitor your breathing intensity. If you are aware of a deeper and more frequent breathing pattern but are not hyperventilating and can still talk to an exercise partner, you are probably exercising within the desired aerobic exercise intensity range.

Finding Your Pulse

Rate of Perceived Exertion Scale	
6	
7	Very, very light
8	
9	Very light
10	
11	Fairly light
12	
13	Somewhat hard
14	
15	Hard
16	
17	Very hard
18	
19	Very, very hard
20	

From Borg, G. "Perceived Exertion: A Note on History and Methods." *Medicine and Science in Sports and Exercise* 5:90–93, 1983.

All about Strength, Function, and Core

Strength is the ability to overcome a resistance. Several studies have shown the health benefits of strength training to include the following:

- ❏ increased metabolic rate
- ❏ increased muscle mass
- ❏ increased bone mineral density
- ❏ improved glucose metabolism
- ❏ improved blood lipid levels
- ❏ reduced lower-back pain
- ❏ reduced arthritic pain
- ❏ improved gastrointestinal transit

Your overall strength is determined by numerous factors, including the intensity of training you regularly do, the predominant muscle fiber type of your muscles, hormonal levels, tendon insertion points, body proportions, and neurological efficiency. Here are some key terms and concepts to know about strength training.

A **concentric muscle action** (or contraction) describes a muscle going through a shortening motion as it overcomes the resistance.

During **eccentric muscle actions** (or contractions), the muscle lengthens as it resists the load. So, if you examine a person doing a biceps curl exercise, the upward phase of the movement is the concentric action, and the lowering phase of the movement is the eccentric action.

An **isometric action** (or contraction) is the amount of strength an individual can exhibit at a single point in the range of motion. With isometric actions, there is no limb movement or change in the joint angle. Just holding a weight in one position is an example of isometric strength.

Speed strength is a new term that is interchangeable with the term power. Speed strength refers to the maximum force exhibited over a distance at a certain speed of movement. Examples of speed strength in sports include swinging a bar, throwing a javelin, and striking a punching bag.

Absolute strength is the maximal amount of weight that an individual can lift at one time. It is sometimes referred to as the one-repetition maximum, abbreviated 1RM.

Relative strength is a useful method for comparing the strength between different individuals. It is the ratio of the amount weight lifted to total body weight. For example, if a person can do a 1RM biceps curl with 50 lbs. and weighs 130 lbs., what is the relative strength for this muscle group? To solve, set up a ratio and compute: 50 lbs./130 lbs. = .38. Relative strength is reported as a percentage, so multiplying by 100 will make this answer 38 percent for the relative strength of the biceps muscles.

Functional strength is a very popular term now used in fitness and sports. In fitness, functional strength applies to doing exercises that will enhance a person's ability to execute everyday activities. Some professionals also use the term **meaningful exercise** to describe functional strength. With functional strength, exercises are chosen that are task specific to help a person perform better in daily life. Numerous exercises throughout this text offer significant functional strength benefits.

In sports, functional strength is used to enhance an athlete's sports performance. For recreational and competitive athletes, trainers and coaches try to duplicate the range of motion (or a portion of the range) with an exercise. For instance, a push-up is excellent for developing the strength of the shoulder joint, yet not the best functional exercise choice for training a golfer. When working with a golfer, the trainer might design an exercise that goes through more of a diagonal pathway, such as the motion of swinging a golf club.

Core strength or core stability training is the newest type of strength training in the health and fitness industry. Core training involves exercises that strengthen the deep spinal muscles. These are the deep abdominal and lower back muscles surrounding the spine, often referred to as the intrinsic muscles. The purpose of core training is to spare the spine from damage. Stability training creates a stable and mobile lower back. Development of core strength leads to a greater enjoyment of exercise participation and improvement in exercise performance. Several exercises in this text have been included to improve core strength.

Muscle hypertrophy literally means an increase in size of muscle. The change in muscle size is reflective of the type and amount of training a person does and is strongly influenced by the amount of muscle-building hormones present, known as androgens.

The Ten Commandments of Strength Training

Doing your exercises is not enough. It's doing them right that really counts. Follow these 10 commandments for effective results.

1. **Control your movement**. Avoid fast, jerky movements that rely too heavily on momentum and may be harmful to your muscles and joints. A safe recommendation for resistance exercise is to perform the ascending motion for two seconds and the descending motion for four seconds.

2. **Perform all exercises through the complete range of motion**. The benefits of strength, endurance, flexibility, skill, and performance are best achieved when exercises are performed through the full range of movement. Sometimes small range-of-motion movements are incorporated with the full range movements. (Exception: to avoid stressing the neck, do not take the head straight back.)

3. **Always exercise opposing muscle groups**. You need to balance the strength of opposing muscles. (See THE MUSCLE SYSTEM for a list of opposing muscle groups.)

4. **Concentrate on the muscles you are working**. Focusing on the specific muscle groups you are working will help you know when and how much to overload.

5. **Do the exercises properly**. The quality, form, and technique of the exercise is very important. Don't just try to see how many repetitions of an exercise you can do!

6. **Breathe normally**. Always exhale as you exert. Do not hold your breath!

7. **Don't exercise to the point of pain**. Pain is a warning sign—STOP before you hurt yourself. For optimal results, challenge yourself to the point of momentary muscular fatigue to sufficiently overload the muscles.

8. **Vary your program and exercises**. This prevents boredom, staleness, and overtraining.

9. **Exercise major body parts early in the workout**. Work your larger muscle groups, such as your legs and chest, before isolating your smaller muscle groups. That way the fatigue in the smaller muscle groups will not affect the performance of the heavier, more-difficult exercises.

10. **Be faithful to your warm-up and cooldown routines**. The warm-up prepares the body for the workout to follow and helps to decrease the risk of injury. It should include low-intensity movements very similar to the workout activity. The cooldown helps the body recover toward a normal resting level. Stretching exercises are recommended to help promote mind and body relaxation and to prevent muscle soreness.

Section 2

Training Tips

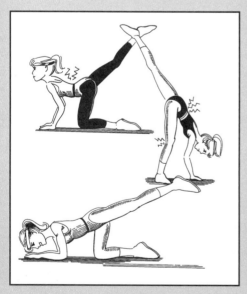

Maximize Your Results, Minimize Your Risks

Not all exercises are good for you. Here are some unsafe or poorly executed exercises with their preferred alternatives.

1. **Twisting Hops** The combination of twisting the spine while hopping on the floor can be quite stressful on the back. The force of hopping alone equals two to three times your body weight.

   Alternative: Jump rope hops do not require any twisting and are more controllable.

2. **Fast-Twisting Waist Exercises** The fast side-to-side twisting of the torso imposes a shearing stress on the vertebrae of the spine.

   Alternative: Do them slowly as a warm-up stretch. Twisting crunches are more effective waist work.

3. **Toe Touches** The straight-legged position stretches the ligaments behind the knees too much and stresses the lower spine. Bouncing touches are even worse!

   Alternative: The seated pike stretch (with slightly bent knees) and the seated half-straddle stretch are much better for you.

4. **Windmill Stretch** This stretch also places too much stress on the ligaments supporting the spine. The twist adds stress to your back.
Alternative: Try a seated side straddle stretch for greater control and safety.

5. **Ballet Barre Leg Stretches** Any person with back problems may inadvertently overstretch the sciatic nerve beyond its normal range.

   Alternative: The single-leg hamstring stretch on the back and the seated half-straddle are recommended alternatives.

6. **Deep Knee Bends** Deep knee bend variations can overstretch the ligaments supporting the knee and compress the cartilage.

   Alternative: When squatting, keep the knees from protruding past the toes, and lower your buttocks to just above your knees.

7. **Lunges with Protruding Knees** The lunge is often incorrectly performed. A bent knee that juts past the ankle places stress on the knee.

   Alternative: Make sure the front knee stays over the toes.

8. **Hurdler's Stretch** This exercise can overstretch the muscles in the groin and the ligaments of the bent knee.

   Alternative: The seated center straddle stretch and half-straddle stretch are better options.

9. **Sit-ups with Straight Legs or Anchored Feet, Double Leg Lifts, Jackknife Sit-ups** These exercises predominantly use the hip flexors (the muscles in front of the thigh that attach to the lower back), not the abdominals! Their repeated performance may lead to back problems.

   Alternative: Use the "crunch" variations that bring your ribs toward your pelvis as you lift only your shoulders and upper back off the floor. See pages 73 and 74.

10. **Head Throws in a Crunch** Often the head is "thrown forward" during a crunch.

    Alternative: Keep your head in a neutral position. Focus on the ceiling.

11. **Swan Lifts** The combination of arching the lower spine as the muscles are contracting can injure the back.

    Alternative: Keep the lower body on the floor and only lift the upper body, as in the back extension. Or, lift one arm in front of the opposite leg in back. Repeat the movement lifting the opposite limbs.

12. **The Plow** This movement places too much stress on the discs and bones of the neck. It may inhibit breathing and blood flow.

    Alternative: The seated pike stretch (with soft knees) is more effective.

13. **Gymnastics Bridges and Pelvic Lifts** The gymnastics bridge, designed to stretch the upper back and shoulders, is usually performed with an overarched lower back. Pelvic lifts are frequently overarched as well.

Alternative: Use the prone prop or prone extension instead of the bridge (See page 43). And be careful not to overarch when performing the pelvic lift.

14. **Leg Lifting Exercises** Leg lifts or side leg exercises can twist and strain the lower back if they are done too fast.

Alternative: Place your elbows on the floor, keep your back straight, and control the movement. Do not swing or fling legs.

15. **Needle Point Exercise** Unless you have great flexibility and control, this places abnormal stress on the lower back and the back of the supporting knee.

Alternative: Regular leg lifts from the elbows and knees are safer and just as effective.

16. **Side Straddle Stretch** If you allow the opposite hip to come off the floor while stretching to the side, you place the hip and spine in poor alignment.

    Alternative: Keep the buttocks and legs firmly on the floor.

17. **Neck Extensions and 360-Degree Head Rolls** Taking the head straight back, as in neck extensions or full head rolls, may place too much stress on the disks of the neck vertebrae.

    Alternative: Neck rotation and lateral flexion are much safer. It is okay to bring the head forward and back, but avoid taking it too far past its neutral position when moving posteriorly.

Twelve Most Common Exercise Mistakes

The following are some of the most common mistakes that occur in exercise programs.

1. **Overtraining** In their zeal to achieve fitness, people often try too hard. Possible signs of overtraining are injury, weight loss, mental dullness, disturbed digestion, loss of appetite, early exhaustion during a workout, fatigue during the day, or elevated heart rate on rising or after a workout. Stress quality, not quantity!

2. **Poor Exercise Technique** Exercises performed incorrectly can lead to injury and poor performance. Poor technique is most frequent during the latter stages of a workout.

3. **Improper Equipment** The exercise clothes you wear, the shoes on your feet, the surface you are training on, and the equipment you are using can all **improve** or **impair** your performance.

4. **Insufficient Warm-up** Too often, the main activity is begun without proper warm-up (or after a quick, insufficient warm-up). This can lead to injury.

5. **Extra-Long Workouts** See signs of overtraining.

6. **Lifting Weights That Are Too Heavy** This leads to improper exercise technique, predisposes you to injury, and is not the progressive overload needed for optimal results in strength and endurance. Realize

your limits.

7. **Forgetting Muscle Groups** For complete body symmetry make sure you work **all** your muscle groups.

8. **Unrealistic Goal Setting** Set realistic short- and long-term goals.

9. **Forced Breathing** Proper breathing during exercise is easy to remember—**exhale** as you **exert.** Do not force your breathing.

10. **Exercises That Are Too Bouncy and Fast** Fast and bouncy movements stimulate your opposing muscle groups to contract and hinder the movement. Control is the key!

11. **Inadequate Aerobic Cooldown** Blood pressure may drop significantly from an abrupt cessation of vigorous aerobic exercise. This may also lead to fainting and irregular heart beats. Slow down gradually; don't just stop!

12. **Insufficient Stretching at the End of the Workout**

Slow stretching following a workout helps reduce muscle soreness and improve flexibility.

Injuries

In Case of Injury

Let's face it, when you pursue an active lifestyle you will occasionally overdo it. And even if you are careful, inadequate equipment (such as poor aerobic shoes) or exercising on an improper surface can lead to injuries. You can usually tell when you have an injury; pain and swelling appear in an area and gradually worsen. What do you do? R.I.C.E. (Rest, Ice, Compression, Elevation) is the answer. Most of these problems are muscle, ligament, and tendon injuries. The R.I.C.E. approach will limit the injury and accelerate the healing.

*R*est: Rest prevents you from reinjury and decreases the circulation to the area. "Time heals."

*I*ce: Ice should be applied immediately to the injured area to keep the swelling down. An ice pack may be applied for 10 to 20 minutes periodically through the first 24 hours. Direct ice massage can be used for 7- to 10-minute sessions with the same effects. Heat can be applied after 48 hours, in conjunction with ice, to increase the circulation and enhance the body's process of removing the excess blood and fluid.

*C*ompression: Compression helps reduce the swelling and internal bleeding. Ace bandages are a good way to do this. Be careful not to obstruct circulation by overtightening!

*E*levation: Elevation helps reduce the internal bleeding and excessive fluid entry to the injury. If possible, elevate the injured area above the level of the heart at all opportune times until the swelling subsides.

See your physician if necessary. Persistent pain, major swelling, and significant discoloration all require elevation. The **cause** of the injury must also be **corrected** so reinjury does not occur. (Maybe you need new shoes, less weight, shorter workouts, etc.) Begin your rehabilitation process of stretching and strengthening and return to your former level of activity when your body is READY!

Common Aerobic Injuries

Shin Splints

The most common aerobic injury is a pain between the knee and ankle, commonly referred to as "shin splints." Shin pain can be caused by a number of conditions, but impact shock is probably the major cause. Rest, ice, and exercise to increase muscle strength/flexibility are standard treatments. Footwear (specifically the arch support), floor surface resiliency, movement selection, and the structure of the workout should be reevaluated for safety and effectiveness. If this pain continues, see your physician.

Knee Injuries

A variety of knee injuries that affect the joint structure may also occur in aerobic exercise. Repeated floor impact and rolling on the foot inward on impact can contribute to these problems. Proper footwear, resilient workout surface, sufficient warm-up, and the progressive increase in exercise intensity will help to prevent these injuries.

Ankle Sprain

An ankle sprain is the most common of all injuries. It usually occurs when the weak ligaments on the outside of the joint are injured by an accidental rolling outward of the ankle. Rest, ice, compression, and elevation are standard treatments; physician referral may be necessary. Safe movement selection, proper warm-up, and concentration on the activity itself will help prevent this type of injury.

Muscle and Ligament Inflammation

Another common injury that occurs from the repeated impact of the foot striking the ground is an inflammation of the muscles and ligaments supporting the foot. Overtraining and improper warm-up often lead to this ailment. Rest, ice, compression, and elevation are recommended treatments. Proper footwear and safe training procedures are preventives.

Guide to a Better Back

It's a pain! Why do you get this lower-back pain and what can you do to prevent back problems? Although there may be a number of different contributing factors to lower-back pain, it's essential to realize that when you stand upright, most of your body weight falls on the lower back. Weak abdominal and back muscles from underuse and/or poor posture may not give the spine the support it needs, leaving the back prone to pain or injury. Your goal to a healthy back is to keep the muscles of the spine, buttocks, and upper legs strong and flexible, be aware of preferred posture, and control your weight.

Healthy Back Tips

Standing and Walking

Maintain your normal back curve, but avoid the swayback posture. Stand tall, feeling lifted throughout the lower abdominal region. Try not to stand still too long. If you must, put one leg up on a support or at least bend alternate knees. Limit your high heel wearing time because these shoes accentuate the back curve and create stress on the spine. Use your abdominal muscles to support your body weight as you stand or move.

Did You Know?

80 percent of Americans encounter a lower-back problem sometime in their daily life.

Lifting

Bend your knees, not your back, when lifting. Hold objects close to your body and avoid over-the-head lifts. Avoid rotating your body when lifting or lowering an object. Instead, change your foot placement while maintaining the object directly in front of you.

Sitting at Your Computer Station

Sit in an adjustable chair that keeps your back upright or slightly forward. The adaptable backrest should maintain your body's natural lower back curve. Your knees should be slightly lower than your hips. Your feet should be firmly placed on the floor or a footrest. Your keyboard should be at elbow level, with the bend at your elbows near 90 degrees. Your hands and wrists should be straight and relaxed. For some people, wrist rests are preferable. Your eyes should be approximately at a midscreen height of your monitor with your head about an arm's length from the screen.

Sleeping

Try sleeping on your side on a firm mattress with your knees slightly bent or on your back with a pillow under your knees. If you must sleep on your stomach, place a small pillow under your abdominals to correct for a sagging spine.

Test Your Posture

With correct posture, you maintain the normal curve in the lower back. Test your posture by standing with your hips, back, and head against the wall. Your heels should be a couple of inches away. There should be only minimal space between your lower back and the wall. You should be standing tall with a long neck and eyes straight forward.

Back Pain Relief

Back injuries require the attention of a specialist. For relief of small aches, lie on your back on a padded surface and elevate your feet (with bent knees) on a padded chair. Place a small pillow or rolled-up towel under your neck and rest in this position for 10 to 15 minutes.

Five Exercises for a Healthy Back

1. **Pelvic Tilt** Lie on your back with knees bent, arms on chest, and feet on floor. Press the lower back into the floor by tightening the abdominal muscles and slightly lifting the buttocks off the floor. Hold for 10 seconds and repeat 8 to 15 times.

2. **Hamstring Stretch** Lie on your back, with both knees bent and one foot on the floor. Grasp behind the lifted knee, bring it toward the chest, and hold for several seconds. Repeat 3 to 5 times on each leg.

3. **Tuck-Hold** Tuck both knees to chest and slowly tighten tuck with arms while you press your lower back into the floor. Keep your back flat. Hold for 15 seconds and repeat 5 to 10 times.

4. **Slow Crunch** Lie on your back with your knees bent at a 45-degree angle and your head supported at the base of the neck by your hands. Slowly lift your chest as you press your lower back into the floor; then slowly lower. Try lifting your buttocks slightly off the floor as you raise the chest. Repeat 8 to 25 times.

5. **Prone Prop** While on your front, lift your chest off the floor and hold by propping your elbows on the ground. Open your legs slightly.

Variation: Same as prone prop, only straighten your arms. For both, relax your hips and abdominals and hold for several seconds and then lower. Repeat 3 to 5 times.

Section 3

Fitness Gear and Where to Train

In Search of the Perfect Aerobic Shoe

The most important investment you can make for aerobics is your shoe. You want a shoe with flexibility, that supports your arches, cushions your heels, adds extra impact absorption at the balls of your feet, and fits well. Here's what to check out:

- ❑ **The outersole** should be flexible, yet durable.

- ❑ **The midsole** (between the outer and inner sole) should provide good stability and cushioning to absorb shock, yet allow for foot flexibility.

- ❑ **The innersole:** A high-shock-absorbent material is recommended. If the shoe you like doesn't have this, purchase an innersole separately.

- ❑ **The toe area:** This is the one place on the shoe where roominess counts. When you exercise, your foot swells. Allow for it. Can you wiggle your toes?

- ❑ **Forefoot cushion:** The greatest amount of force the foot must absorb is behind the ball of the foot. There must be good cushioning here.

- ❑ **Forefoot flexibility:** The shoe should bend (as the foot does) at the ball of the foot. Too stiff a forefoot will cause lower leg discomfort. This area needs to be flexible yet stable.

- ❑ **Arch support:** Make sure the arch provides comfortable support.

- ❑ **The heel counter:** This should be an inflexible material surrounding the heel area, holding it in place. The more it prevents excessive rolling and twisting, the better it is.

- ❑ **The shoe heel:** Look for an outer heel that makes a flush contact with the ground. If the inner heel height is too low, it will cause an excessive pull on the calf and Achilles tendon. The heel should provide good cushion without being too hard or too soft. Shoes are now designed in high-top ankle support. These help out a lot.

- ❑ **Comfort:** Try them on in the store and move around for 10 minutes. Don't purchase them if they feel uncomfortable. Also, because your feet swell during the day, it is best to purchase shoes in the afternoon or evening.

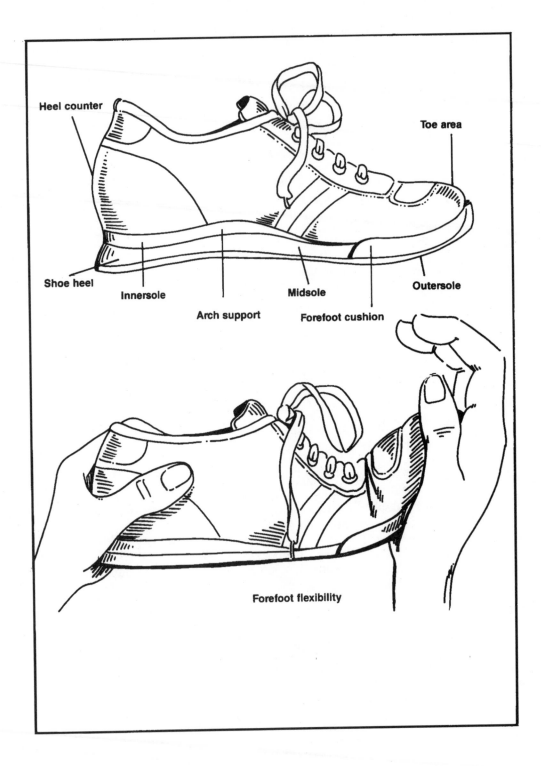

Heel counter

Toe area

Shoe heel

Innersole

Midsole

Outersole

Arch support

Forefoot cushion

Forefoot flexibility

How to Choose a Health Club

Try to visit the prospective health club during the time you would be using the facility. Shop around, using the following as a helpful checklist.

1. Is the location convenient to your home, work, or school?

2. Is it a workout gym, a social club, a coed facility, or a fitness center for families? What are you looking for?

3. Does the facility look clean, organized, seasonally air-controlled, and suitably lighted? Specifically check out the locker room and showers for cleanliness!

4. What facilities should you look for?

   ❑ Well-equipped exercise rooms with top equipment. Are there enough weight-resistance machines, stationary bikes, treadmills, rowing machines, free weights, and space to accommodate the members?

   ❑ An aerobic exercise room with a proper floor. Does it have a floating wood design or is it carpet, wood, or linoleum over cement (which is much more unsafe)? Does it have enough space for the class sizes? Is it air-conditioned?

   ❑ Accessible racquetball or squash courts. What is the court reservation procedure? (If you have to reserve over 48 hours in advance, you know that they are getting heavy use.) Do the court floors and walls look very marked up? Do you have to pay for court time?

   ❑ Well-maintained pool. Is it heated year-round? Is the size suitable to your needs?

   ❑ Available track facilities. Is there an indoor or outdoor track?

   ❑ Relaxing spa facilities. Is there a whirlpool, sauna, steam room, massage room, and cold plunge?

   ❑ Well-kept locker room. Do you get a locker and key every time you use the facility? Or do you bring your own lock or rent out the locker? Does the club provide towels, soap, shampoo, hair dryers, and other grooming amenities?

5. What kind of staff does it have? Are there any trained personnel in physical education, exercise physiology, nutrition, or sports medicine? Does the staff have a professional, friendly, and helpful attitude?

6. What type of programs do they run? Are there enough classes in a variety of workouts? Are there additional fees? Can you take a class any time you wish?

7. Do the club hours fit your needs?

8. **Examine the fees carefully!**

   ☐ Are they affordable? Is there a payment plan?

   ☐ Is there an initiation fee? Is it refundable? Is this a one-time charge or a yearly charge? Are there any monthly dues in addition? How much?

   ☐ Be leery of contracts and "too good to be true" promotionals. Read all the small print before you sign.

   ☐ Be wary of "lifetime" memberships—is it your lifetime or the club's?

   ☐ What are the cancellation policies? Must you sell your membership? Do you get a pro-rated refund?

   ☐ Read with caution any "preopening" sales packages.

9. Does the club allow you to put your membership on hold for a short period (such as for a vacation) without having to pay the monthly dues?

10. How much does it cost to bring a guest to the club? Does the club give out guest passes?

11. How long has the club been in operation?

12. How long has the present management been with the club?

13. Ask if the club belongs to any national trade organization with an established code of ethics for staff and clients.

14. Before joining, talk to some members as they enter or on leaving the facility to get their opinions of the club.

Creating a Home Gym

You don't have to be rich to create a convenient home gym. Even if you belong to a club or studio, your schedule or occasional desire for workout privacy may warrant the purchase of home exercise equipment. Here are some tips to get you started.

1. Make sure you have enough space. A wall mirror helps you view your exercise technique and serves as a great motivator. Music helps too!

2. Make sure the lighting and air ventilation are adequate.

3. Before purchasing any equipment, identify your fitness needs. Do you want a jump rope, treadmill, stationary cycle, rowing machine, or step for cardiorespiratory fitness? Do you want equipment for specific exercises for your abdominals, legs, and buttocks? Having identified your fitness needs will prevent you from purchasing equipment of no value to you.

4. Look for equipment that features effective safety measures and provides progressive exercise guidelines.

5. Shop around. It's amazing how the cost of the same equipment varies from store to store! Examine the warranty and service agreements closely.

6. Watch out for attractive, shiny, lightweight equipment that lacks durability and stability.

7. Try the equipment out. Not all equipment feels the same. With mail-order equipment, review the return policies and procedures carefully before purchasing. Are the shipping charges reasonable?

8. Build your exercise area to fit your program. Buy a little at a time and add as you see fit.

9. Stay away from products that guarantee phenomenal results in a short time.

10. When purchasing equipment on sale, see if the product is being discontinued. If it is, there may be a newer, better style available at the same price.

11. For display purposes, store equipment is usually free standing and movable. Check to see which products need to be firmly secured to a wall or floor, and how they need to be secured.

Finding the Right Instructor

All instructors have their own teaching style, and classes have their own special characteristics. Here's what to look for in an instructor and class to make sure it meets your needs.

1. Take a trial class or observe the instructor and class during the time you would normally attend.

2. Look for **quality** and not **quantity.** Just because a class does numerous repetitions or the instructor is "tough" doesn't mean it's a good class.

3. Does the instructor make an effort to teach, correct, explain, and give clear directions? Can you hear the verbal instructions? Does the instructor modify exercises for the students who have special needs?

4. If there is a mirror, does the instructor face it throughout most of the class? Mirrors are wonderful instructional aids, but direct eye contact is one of the most effective means of communication and interaction.

5. Look for a well-rounded workout: a thorough warm-up, a gradually building aerobic section, a winding down of the aerobics, a complete body firming section, and a cool-down stretching segment.

6. Does the workout seem to flow smoothly from one section to the next?

7. Is the class easy to follow? Could you see the instructor easily or was it too crowded?

8. Does the instructor inspire and motivate you? Did you enjoy the workout?

9. Was the workout challenging enough for you? Does the club or studio offer a variety of different levels and styles of classes?

10. Did you feel comfortable with the class atmosphere?

11. Could you hear the music? Was it too loud?

12. What training, credentials, and education does the instructor have? The credibility of an instructor who boasts of "being certified" cannot always be substantiated. Inquire about any specific training, experience, and education the instructor has had.

13. Does the class follow a prescribed exercise program? The American College of Sports Medicine recommends aerobic activity three to five times a week for between 20 and 60 minutes, at 55 percent to 90 percent of your maximum heart rate.

14. Is there any type of medical screening for participants prior to participation?

15. Is the cost of the class or program within your budget?

16. Is the class in a convenient location?

Section 4

Let's
Work Out

Warm up First

Let's get ready for the movement to follow and prevent any injuries!

Warm-up Do's and Don'ts	
Do's	**Don'ts**
Move slowly and rhythmically.	Bounce, jerk or force positions.
Focus on full-body range of motion.	"Lock" your joints.
Perform all warm-up exercises on both sides.	

First off: Active Start

Begin with three to five minutes of **easy** aerobics, brisk walking, or cycling to elevate the body temperature, stimulate circulation to the muscles, and loosen up the joints to prepare them for more strenuous exercise.

Then, try the following series of warm-up exercises:

Head
(For neck)

Action: Take head from one side, forward, and around to other side. Reverse. Also, turn head from side to side.

Tips: Avoid taking the head to a straight back position. Make sure these movements are performed slowly.

Shoulder Rolls
(For shoulders)

Action: Smooth circles with shoulders (arms down at side).

Tips: Circle in both directions.

Torso Side Stretch
(For side and hips)

Action: Reach one arm over your head and stretch your torso sideways. Stretch other side. Keep the knees slightly bent.

Tips: Be sure to face forward so you don't twist as you stretch. Support yourself with your extended arm on the thigh to avoid spinal stress.

Torso Twist
(For spine)

Action: Twist gently and rhythmically from the waist.

Tips: Keep your knees slightly bent and control the movement.

Arm Reaches
(For upper back)

Action: Reach with alternating arms over the head, lengthening the upper torso.

Tips: Keep your weight evenly balanced with your lower body. Look up slightly as you do your reaches.

Lunge Stretch: High and Low
(For thighs and lower leg)

Action: Bend front knee and keep back leg straight.
High Lunge: Stretch the Achilles tendon and calf by gently bending and straightening the back leg.
Low Lunge: Stretch the hips down into the floor. Other side.

Tips: Keep the front knee over the ankle and the toes pointing forward.

Upper Spine/Shoulder Stretch

Action: Place hands on thighs above knees. Keep your knees bent. Press one shoulder down and allow the trunk and head to rotate, stretching the upper back, shoulder, and neck. To other side.

Tips: Always keep your knees slightly bent and do not bend over too far forward.

Aerobics: The Main Event

Following are some aerobic steps you can perform to lively music. Start gradually at a brisk walking pace, increase your intensity into your target zone, and then wind back down to a brisk walk. To improve your aerobic efficiency, build up to 20 continuous minutes, three to five times a week. Be creative and "choreograph" your own routines! You can create variety by using various arm positions, lifting your legs to different heights, adding a clap, and traveling in a circle or in different directions. Also, all aerobic skills can be modified by just bending and lifting the legs without "bouncing" on the floor. This is called "low-impact" aerobics. A combination of "low-impact" with "impact" aerobics is recommended to reduce the potential of overuse injuries on the body's lower extremities.

Aerobic Reminders

❏   Wear good aerobic shoes.

❏   Listen to your body.

❏   Check your heart rate and perceived exertion focusing on breathing intensity and the talk test.

❏   Go at your own pace.

❏   Make floor contact with your whole foot.

❏   Do not hop on one foot more than four times in a row.

❏   Stay away from twisting hop variations (stress on the spine). Drink water during exercise; your thirst doesn't keep up with your body's need for water.

❏   Important: gradually wind down your aerobics to a brisk walking pace. This is called the aerobic cooldown.

JOGGING IN PLACE

STEP KNEE HOPS

STEP KICKS

SIDE
LEG
SLIDES

JUMP
ROPE
HOPS

POWER RUNS

SKI HOPS

JUMPING JACKS

LUNGE CLAPS

JUMP
← KICKS →

STRIDE
RUNS

Stepping Up

Stepping is a very popular group exercise activity. It offers a considerable amount of variety to aerobic exercise classes while contributing to the concept of cross-training. The recognized originator of this famously popular exercise activity discovered it accidentally. While doing knee rehabilitation exercises on a bench, this aerobic professional noted that it could be made much more enjoyable if done to music with a little movement creativity. Fitness professionals and enthusiasts worldwide are the fortunate recipients of this person's inventive contribution to fitness.

Stepping can best be described as a low-impact activity capable of providing high-intensity aerobic conditioning for the participant. The workout can be as challenging as vigorous jogging and yet produce impact forces as safe as walking. The feeling of this activity is very similar to the workout you get from climbing stairs. The cadence of the stepping is slower than the movement tempos you would use in an aerobic class (approximately 118 to 126 beats per minutes), because of the greater ranges of motion offered by the platform and because of a concern for safety.

Steps range in height from 4 inches to 12 inches and have a stepping surface of 14 inches wide and up to 4 feet long. It is recommended that you begin gradually, using a lower height step, and progressively increase toward higher step platforms as you become more capable of handling the challenging work. Step workouts are excellent additions to the other aerobic workouts you enjoy doing.

I have presented the basic steps and patterns for you to learn on your step. Treat this workout like any other workout. You need to warm up your body the same as prescribed in the warm-up section. Devote a little more time to warm up the ankles for a step training workout. Accompany this workout with specific body sculpturing exercises of your choice, and don't forget your cooldown stretches at the end of the workout. Each step is most easily categorized by the direction in which the body faces the platform. The specific directions include:

❑ From the front

❑ From the side

❑ From a straddle stand

❑ From the top

❑ From the end

Each step is further classified as either a basic or single lead step where the same foot leads every cycle, or as an alternating step where the lead step alternates every four counts. When doing a single lead step, a good rule to follow is to lead with the same leg for no more than 1 minute before changing to the other foot. When doing an alternating lead step, a good rule to follow is to continue the step for no longer than 2 minutes. What about arm choreography? Focus on learning the basic steps at first. Arm choreography will come naturally as you become more comfortable with your stepping patterns.

Here are some basic moves to get you stepping.

Basic Step

a. **Directional approach:** From the front.

b. **Performance:** Right foot up, left foot up, right foot down, left foot down, and continue. (Do on both sides.)

c. **Pattern:** Up, up, down, down.

Alternating Basic Step

a. **Directional approach:** From the front.

b. **Performance:** Right foot up, left foot up, right foot down, left foot down (tap), switch lead to left foot up, right foot up, left foot down, right foot down (tap) switch lead, and continue.

c. **Pattern:** Up, up, down, tap, up, up, down, tap.

Basic V-Step

a. **Directional approach:** From the front.

b. **Performance:** Right foot up and out, left foot up and out, right foot down, left foot down, and continue. (Do on both sides.)

Performance Tip: Step with a wide V pattern by opening the legs on top of the platform and bringing them together on the floor.

c. **Pattern:** Up, up, down, down.

d. **Variation:** Can also do with an alternating basic step pattern.

Alternating Knee-up Step

a. **Directional approach:** From the front.

b. **Performance:** Right foot up, left knee up, left foot down, right foot down. Left foot up, right knee up, right foot down, left foot down. Continue pattern.

c. **Pattern:** Up, knee, down, down; up other knee, down, down.

Across the Top Step

a. **Directional approach:** From the side.

b. **Performance:** Right foot up, left foot up, right foot down, left foot down (tap), switch to left foot up, right foot up, left foot down, right foot down (tap). Continue the alternating across the top pattern.

c. **Pattern:** Up, across, down, tap; up, across, down, tap.

Straddle Down Step

a. **Directional approach:** From the top.

b. **Performance:** Right foot down on side of platform, left foot down on side of platform, right foot up, left foot up. (Do on both sides.)

c. **Pattern:** Down, down, up, up.

d. **Variation:** Can also do with an alternating step pattern.

Straddle Up Step

a. **Directional approach:** From a straddle stand.

b. **Performance:** Right foot up, left foot up, right foot down, left foot down. (Do on both sides.)

c. **Pattern:** Up, up, down, down.

d. **Variation:** Can also do with an alternating step pattern.

Alternating Straddle Knee Lift Step

a. **Directional approach:** From a straddle stand.

b. **Performance:** Right foot up, left knee lift, left foot down to floor, right foot down to floor. Left foot up, right knee lift, right knee down to floor, left foot down to floor. Continue the alternating knee lift pattern.

c. **Pattern:** Up, knee lift, down, down; Up, knee lift, down, down.

Alternating Side Lunge Step

a. **Directional approach:** From the top.

b. **Performance:** Right foot down and out, right foot on top of platform; left foot down and out, left foot on top of platform. Continue alternating from side to side.

c. **Pattern:** Lunge out, up, lunge out, up.

From the End Step

a. **Directional approach:** From the end.

b. **Performance:** Use the end of the platform to combine several of the steps introduced earlier for variety.

Stepping Safety

1. **Make sure you step entirely on the top part of the platform with each step, not allowing any part of your foot to hang over the edge.**

2. **Start with a 4 inch or 6 inch height.** Don't rush to raise the height of the bench. Most people find the 6" height to provide a satisfactory workout. The recommendation to avoid flexing the knee more than 90 degrees with your step height is a conservative guideline that is easy to follow.

3. **Adding handheld weights (up to 4 lbs.) changes your arm choreography to slow, controlled, nonrotational, shorter-lever movements.**

4. **Stop stepping and march in place on the ground whenever you want to lower the intensity.**

5. **Be careful not to step too far back off the platform.** This causes the body to lean slightly forward, placing extra stress on the Achilles tendon and calf.

6. **Use a good cross-training shoe or indoor fitness shoe for your workout.** The tread on some running shoes does not provide suitable freedom of movement or support.

7. **Step onto and off the platform.** Avoid pounding your feet on the ground and platform. Also, try not to step with a bounce; this causes you to remain the balls of your feet.

8. **Remember not to lock your knees on the descending phase of the step pattern.**

9. **Avoid any movements that travel forward and down off the bench.**

10. **Drink plenty of water, as you tend to sweat a little more with step training.**

11. **Be aware of the potential for overuse injury syndrome.** Many people will enjoy the variety and uniqueness of step training so much that they will discontinue their other physical activities. Doing a variety of exercise programs lessens the stress on many specific body parts, and still allows you to place a lot of demands on your body.

12. **If you feel any discomfort underneath or around the knee you need to stop.** See your health practitioner. Bench stepping may not be the best activity for you.

13. **Always watch your platform when stepping, but don't drop the head forward.** Also, move your arms through low, mid, and high ranges of motion.

14. **As you step, avoid unnecessary forward bending at the hips.** This may put too much stress on your back.

15. **Be careful of overusing the lunge skills.** They can cause you to lean too far forward, stressing your lower back, and they can place extra joint trauma on the lower leg with ground impact.

16. **Change the leading foot of your stepping patterns regularly to avoid over-stressing one leg.** A good rule of thumb is to not lead with one leg for more than a minute.

17. **To avoid stress on the leg, do not perform more than five consecutive repeating movements on the same leg.**

Aerobic Kickboxing: A Knockout Punch

Aerobic kickboxing, kickbox fitness, box-step and cardio-karate are a few class names that have become a staple core of the group-led exercise industry. Enthusiasts are enjoying the power from throwing kicks, punches, elbows, jabs, knee strikes, and combinations used in boxing and kickboxing. The athletic drills in these classes are mixed with recovery bouts of basic aerobic movements such as boxer-style rope skipping and easy jogging. Some programs utilize authentic boxing and martial arts equipment whereas others do a form of "shadow boxing." All classes are driven by high-energy music and have provided a new alternative to group-led exercise classes, which appeal to both women and men. Research from this author suggests that the energy cost of this type of exercise ranges from 6.5 to 8.4 kilocalories a minute for a 130-pound female.

With the popularity and excitement however, some new challenges have surfaced such as safety for the participants. A key concern is that instructors have the proper knowledge to teach correct punching techniques. The challenge involves integrating skill with a motivating workout environment. Several organizations have established their own standards of safety, but there are no nationally accepted guidelines among certifying groups. The best advice to participants is to make sure the class instructor has had some type of specialized training and/or certification. Instructors need to be aware of the appropriate development skills and precautions to use when teaching these martial arts workouts.

Body Conditioning Workouts

Four different body conditioning programs follow for your toning workouts. They are:

1. Site-specific exercise section for distinctive body areas.

2. Super sculpturing program with hand weights.

3. Circuit training course with complete instructions on how to progressively overload the program.

4. Power sculpturing exercises and workout.

For best body shaping results, regularly vary your selection of these workouts to constantly challenge your muscles.

Chest, Shoulder, and Arm Developers

Perform 10 to 30 repetitions of each exercise.

Modified or Regular Push-ups
(Chest, shoulders, and arms)

Action: Lower torso all the way to the floor and up.

Tips: Keep the back straight.

Wide-Arm Push-ups
(Chest and arms)

Action: Same as push-up with arms placed beyond shoulder width. Open legs to a straddle position.

Tips: Make sure fingers are pointed away from body.

Pike Push-ups
(Shoulders and triceps—back of the arms)

Action: A push-up with hips up and hands closer to feet. Legs together or open to a straddle.

Tips: Placing the hands closer together is more challenging.

Dips
(Shoulders, chest, and triceps)

Action: With hands by side on chair or floor, bend and extend arms.

Tips: Hands should face forward. Keep legs extended when using chair.

For a Stable Core: The Excellent Eight

Perform 15 to 40 repetitions of each exercise.

Regular Crunch
(Abdominals)

Action: Lift the back and shoulders off the floor. Push the small of the back against the floor. Rotate pelvis so buttocks are slightly off floor.

Tips: Feet are on the floor approximately six to ten inches from the buttocks. Hands may support the head at the base of the neck or lie across the chest. Focus on the ceiling.

Variation: Squeeze your knees together for inner thigh work as well.

Twisting Crunch
(Abdominals and obliques—sides)

Action: Alternate shoulders as you lift your upper back off the floor.

Tips: Vary your technique by either lifting first and then twisting or by twisting first and then lifting.

Reverse Crunch
(Lower abdominals)

Action: Slowly lift buttocks off the ground a couple of inches.

Tips: Keep the knees bent.

Variation: Bring chest toward knee (as you lift the buttocks) for an even more challenging crunch. Press the heels into the buttocks to relax your hip flexors and work the abdominals more.

Rope Pull Crunch
(Abdominals and obliques)

Action: Lift shoulder blades off the floor and alternate reaching the arms (as if pulling a rope).

Tips: Make sure the small of the back is pressed into floor.

The All-Around Crunch
(Abdominals and obliques)

Action: Alternate with a twisting crunch to one side, a regular crunch straight up, and a twisting crunch to the other side.

Tips: Lift the legs so the thighs are perpendicular to the floor and bent at the knees. You may wish to place your feet on a chair.

Variation: Randomly mix the pattern of the side, up, other side to surprise your abdominal muscles—they have to work harder!

Back Extension
(After working the abdominal muscles, it is correct to work the opposite muscle group: the lower back.)

Action: Slowly lift the head, shoulders, and chest off the floor from the prone position. The arms may help with the lift, remain at the sides, or be held close to the shoulders.

Tips: Keep the feet on the floor to protect the spine. Stretch up and out.

Horizontal Side Bridge
(Deep abdominals and spinal muscles)

Action: Do this exercise on a padded surface. Lie on your side with the knees bent at about a 90-degree angle. With the abdominals pulled in, push up with the elbow, lifting the torso off the ground. Hold for 6 seconds and then lower and repeat several times on both sides.

Tips: Keep the nonsupportive hand on the opposite shoulder.

Variation: For greater challenge, do the exercise with the knees off the floor and legs extended.

Rolling Side Bridge
(Deep abdominals and spinal muscles)

Action: Lie on your side with your legs extended. Pull in the abdominal muscles and push up to a side bridge. Roll slowly to a front prone position with both elbows on the ground and then roll to the other elbow.

Tips: Move very slowly and work up to repeating this entire sequence for up to 30 seconds or until the muscles fatigue.

Variation: For a more challenging side bridge, place the upper foot in front of the lower foot. This will cause more instability, making you work your intrinsic spinal muscles even more.

Thighs, Hips, and Buttocks

These body parts are best worked together! Use elastic resistance or exercise equipment or wear leg weights for an adequate overload. Perform 15 to 30 repetitions of each exercise.

Back Thigh Lifts
(Back thigh, buttocks, and hip)

Action: Keeping an erect standing position with the resistance on one ankle, bring the leg toward the rear to a comfortable ending point.

Tips: For balance, place one arm on an immobile surface.

Variation: Do this exercise slightly toward the angle (between straight back and to the side). It works the same muscles and some people find it more comfortable.

Hip Adduction
(Inner thigh)

Action: From a standing position, extend one leg to the side making sure you feel a moderate resistance on the leg. Pull the leg in front and across the midline of the body. Return slowly to starting position.

Tips: Try not to let the body twist during this exercise.

Variation: Hold leg across midline of movement for 3 seconds before returning to starting position.

Hip Abduction
(Outer thighs and hips)

Action: From a standing position with feet together and resistance strap around the outer leg, lift the leg straight to the side.

Tips: Do not let the body swing from side to side and keep your feet facing forward.

Variation: Hold the movement for 3 seconds out to the side before returning to starting position.

Bird-Dog Exercise
(Buttocks and lower back)

Action: Starting on the hands and knees, slowly raise one arm and the opposite leg to a horizontal position and hold for 6 seconds. Lower the arm and leg and then repeat with the other arm and opposite leg. Repeat several times.

Tips: Pull in the abdominals while doing this exercise.

Variation: You can also do this exercise while lying in a prone position.

Tightening Tips

- ❑ Remember to repeat all exercises on both sides. Vary your exercise performance tempo.
- ❑ There is a tendency in leg work to roll back at the hip and let the powerful quadriceps (front of the thigh muscles) do the work—watch your technique.
- ❑ It is not necessary to lift the legs high for results.
- ❑ Combine full range-of-motion exercises with "pulse" movements—take the leg to the top end of the range and perform small "pulse" movements.

Inner Thigh Extras

Inner Thigh Lifts—Knee Down

Action: Lie on side with head supported by bent arm or resting on straight arm. Bring top leg over extended bottom leg and relax top knee into the floor. Lift lower leg up and down.

Tips: Concentrate on lifting with bottom heel. Perform 15 to 30 repetitions.

Inner Thigh Lifts—Knee Up

Action: Same as above. Place top leg over bottom leg with foot in front of knee. Lift lower leg up and down.

Tips: Concentrate on lifting with bottom heel. Perform 15 to 30 repetitions.

Wide Squats

Action: Stand with feet placed wider than shoulders. Keeping your back straight, bend your knees until your buttocks are slightly above knee height. Hold this position for 15 to 30 seconds.

Tips: Make sure your knees point directly over your toes.

Variation: While in this squat position go up and down very slowly and focus on using the muscles of the inner thigh.

Super Sculpturing with Weights

If you really want to attain that sleek, firm, and shapely look, use weights. You can work all the major muscles of the body with hand weights. Perform 8 to 20 repetitions of each exercise, doing two to four sets of each exercise. Be sure to rest 30 to 60 seconds between sets.

Squat
(Buttocks and thighs)

Action: Stand with feet placed wider than shoulders. Hold weights into chest or next to shoulders. Keeping your back straight, bend legs and squat down with your buttocks no lower than your knee height and return to start.

Tips: Make sure your buttocks go back as you sit and your knees stay over your toes. Do this carefully if you have knee problems!

Variation: Change the width of your stance to work all the muscles completely.

Long Lunge
(Thighs and buttocks)

Action: Stand with feet together and hand weights next to shoulder or down by your side. Step forward about two to three feet with one leg to a bent knee position. Keep the back leg extended, allowing it to bend slightly. Push back to a stand and repeat on other leg.

Tips: Keep your back straight and press into the bending leg.

Variation: Stand with feet together and hand weights by side. "Step back" into lunge position.

Short Lunge
(Thighs and buttocks)

Action: Stand with one foot two to three feet in front of the other foot. Hold weights next to your sides. Bend both legs so the back knee comes within six inches of the ground and then straighten up. Do on both sides.

Tips: Turn toes out slightly for balance.

Heel Raises
(Calves)

Action: Stand with legs wider than shoulder width, feet slightly turned out. Hold weights along sides. Lift heels high off the ground and then lower.

Tips: Perform this exercise on a thick book or block of wood to allow a larger range of motion.

Chest Press
(Chest, shoulders, and arms)

Action: Lie on a bench or floor with hand weights held by shoulders. Extend arms straight up and back down to side.

Tips: Keep elbows out from body at the start for effective chest overload. Bend knees with feet on the bench (ground) or with knees pulled toward the chest to safeguard the lower back.

Flys
(Chest and arms)

Action: Same position (on bench or floor) as chest press. Start with hand weights extended above chest and lower arms perpendicularly away from body and then back up.

Tips: Keep arms slightly bent throughout the exercise and palms facing each other.

Variation: Modify the position of the hand weights as they extend over the chest.

Crunches with Weights
(Abdominals)

Action: With back on the floor, weight(s) held behind the head or on the chest, lift upper back off the floor and lower. Lower legs placed on a chair.

Tips: Press the small of the back into the floor.

Variation: Twist side to side in the crunch.

Standing Rows
(Upper and middle back)

Action: Stand in a straddle position with head up and upper body slightly forward. Hand weights are extended in front of body. Pull elbows as far back as they will go and return to start.

Tips: Do not bend forward too much (this may stress the spine).

Variation: Stand in lunge position with weight in one hand. Bend over at waist and place other hand on bent knee for support. Pull arm straight back and lower.

Shoulder Press
(Shoulders and triceps)

Action: May be done standing or sitting.

Shoulder: Start with hand weights held next to shoulder. Press weights straight over head and return to start.

Tips: Make sure you keep your back stable during the exercise.

Variation: Alternate pressing one arm and then the other arm to concentrate on each side.

Side Lateral Raises
(Shoulders and back)

Action: Hold hand weights next to your side. Keeping arms slightly bent, elevate weights laterally to shoulder height and lower.

Tips: Do not "lock" elbow joints or raise arms above shoulders.

Variation: For more upper back work, sit in a chair and bend forward at hips. Lift weights to shoulder height with bent arms and lower.

Tricep Extensions
(Triceps—back of arms)

Action: Stand with legs shoulder-width apart and knees bent. Bring weights up, bending elbows up and back. From this position, extend arms straight back and then return to start.

Tips: Keep the elbows from swinging forward and back.

Variation: Extend elbows to the side and open arms to the side (no higher than shoulders).

Bicep Curls

(Biceps—front of arms)

Action: Stand with legs shoulder-width apart and knees bent. Bring weights to shoulder and lower.

Tips: Keep the hands in a "palm-up" position.

Variation: Alternate lifting one arm and then the other. Or do the curls in a lunge position.

Super Sculpture Tips

❑ Find a hand weight that's comfortable, yet challenging.

❑ For variety, vary the number of repetitions, the sequence of exercises, the number of sets, or the weight.

❑ For best results perform this routine two or (preferably) three times a week.

❑ As the weight gets easy to work with, gradually overload with a heavier weight, more repetitions, more sets, or less time between sets.

❑ Try a circuit training format (time effective and good for muscular endurance training): perform a set of each exercise and then move to the next exercise without resting. Perform two to four circuits.

❑ Refer to *A Circuit Workout* for more on circuit training.

A Circuit Workout

SHOULDER PRESS

SQUATS

START

FINISH

Circuit training is one of the most popular forms of training because you constantly move and change from one exercise to another. No rest is needed between exercises because you are working different muscle groups at each station. Circuit training can be performed with or without weights. By placing an aerobic station between each exercise (except for those done lying on the floor), you can burn additional calories and improve your level of fitness.

WIDE-ARMED PUSH-UPS

BIRD-DOG EXERCISE

BACK EXTENSIONS

POWER LUNGES

SIDE LATERAL RAISES

Perform 15 to 30 repetitions at each station for a 45-second work interval. Then move to the next station. Go through the circuit two to three times. Try working out to music. Make sure you warm up before you start and stretch out when you finish. You can progressively overload by the following means (but choose only one method at a time):

1. Increase the number of stations.

2. Repeat the circuit another time.

3. Increase the number of repetitions at each station.

4. Increase the load of weights.

5. Increase the pace of the workload.

STANDING ROWS

BICEP CURLS

CRUNCHES   **TRICEP EXTENSIONS**

Power Sculpturing Exercise

The following "power" exercises are original movement combinations biomechanically designed to effectively challenge the body. This program will offer creativity while improving your functional strength and core stability. Begin with a comfortable starting weight and gradually overload with heavier resistance. For variety, perform the standing power exercises in random order, changing movements after every eight repetitions. Do all movements with control.

Power Side

(Abductors, adductors, gluteals, quadriceps, hamstrings, deltoids, triceps)

Action: From a wide squat, extend legs lifting one leg off the ground as you straighten your arms. Return to squat and alternate sides.

Tips: Keep the lifting leg from rotating outward to effectively work the abductors. On all squats, be sure to keep the buttocks at or above standing knee height.

Power Ski

(Abductors, adductors, gluteals, quadriceps, hamstrings, deltoids, pectorals)

Action: From a wide squat, extend legs to lift and flex one leg as you squeeze your elbows together. Return to wide squat and alternate sides.

Tips: Make sure you lift your knee to the side. Keep legs slightly wider than shoulder width in all wide squats.

Power Knee

(Quadriceps, gluteals, hip flexors, deltoids, triceps)

Action: From a narrow squat position with legs close together, extend legs, lifting one leg with a bent knee as you extend the arms over the head. Lower to narrow squat and alternate sides.

Tips: Keep your back straight and the buttocks back as you sit in a narrow squat. Do not go as low in the narrow squat as you do in the wide squat.

Power Deltoid
(Adductors, quadriceps, gluteals, hamstrings, deltoids)

Action: Extend your legs from a squat as you laterally raise your arms to shoulder height. Lower and repeat.

Tips: Raise and lower your arms (with control) making sure to keep them shoulder height or below in the top position.

Power Row
(Spinal extensors, quadriceps, gluteals, hamstrings, trapezius)

Action: Extend your body and legs from a flexed squat position as you lift your elbows above your head.

Tips: Keep your hands close together, stopping them under your chin at the top position. To effectively work the spinal extensors, you need to find a comfortable yet challenging starting position where the trunk is flexed. Keep the head up and the back straight.

Power Lunge
(Quadriceps, hamstrings, gluteals, biceps)

Action: From a standing position with arms by your side, step back into a lunge position and perform a bicep curl with your arms. Return to the starting position and repeat on other side.

Tips: Be sure to keep your bent knee over your ankle and your weight forward.

Variations: Turn your knuckles toward your shoulders and perform a reverse arm curl. You can also vary the degree of difficulty by keeping your knees slightly bent throughout the exercise.

Power Hamstring
(Hamstrings)

Action: Stand with one leg three feet in front of the other leg with the toes facing forward. Hold weights down by sides. With your weight supported over your front leg, bend the back leg bringing the heel toward the buttocks and then lower the leg to the floor. Complete repetitions on one leg before switching sides. As the back leg bends, bring the arms up along the torso.

Tips: Do not allow the knee of the working leg to come forward. As you curl the leg, keep the upper body stable to support the lower back.

Power Hip
(Gluteals, hamstrings, triceps)

Action: Stand with one leg three feet behind the other leg and slightly out to the side. Bring the weights just under the shoulders. Lift the back leg toward the diagonal plane. Lower leg slowly to floor. As the leg goes back diagonally, the arms extend out to the side and return as the leg lowers to floor. Complete repetitions on one leg before switching sides.

Tips: Squeeze the buttocks as you lift and lower the leg. Try to do the action with a smooth rhythm throughout the range.

Power Sculpturing Workout

Following is a recommended sequence of exercises for a muscular endurance workout. You will effectively work your body's muscular system, progressing from larger (more energy demanding) muscle groups to smaller (more specific) muscles. To overload, vary the number of repetitions, the number of sets, the movement tempo, or the weight. Perform exercises half-time using music with 140 to 150 beats per minute.

- ❑ **Standing Power Moves:** Power side, power ski, power knee, power row, power deltoid, power lunge, power hamstring, power hip

- ❑ **Gastrocnemius/Anterior Tibialis:** Heel raises with feet facing out, forward, and in; toe lifts for anterior tibialis

- ❑ **Pectorals:** Standing flys with bent arms (arms high and low), chest/elbow squeezes

- ❑ **Rhomboids/Trapezius:** Standing row, single arm row, reverse fly (standing or with one knee on the floor)

- ❑ **Abdominals:** Crunch, twisting crunch, rope pull crunch, all-around crunch, reverse crunch (all abdominal exercises with or without hand weights)

- ❑ **Specific Gluteals, Abductors, Adductors:** Prone leg lifts, outer leg lifts, inner thigh lifts

- ❑ **Deltoids:** Shoulder press (in seated position)

- ❑ **Triceps/Deltoid/Chest:** Wide-arm push-ups, pike push-ups, triceps extension on knees (or seated)

- ❑ **Biceps:** Bicep curls and alternating arm bicep curls

Stability Ball Training

Originating from Europe, stability ball training is spreading throughout the United States. Although originally used in rehabilitation, stability ball training is now used in group-led exercise classes and by home fitness buffs. These round, beach-ball-looking devices provide an unstable base for exercises to be performed. The unstable nature of the ball allows more muscles to be challenged when performing exercises on or with the stability ball. Ball size is quite variable; however, a good rule of thumb when selecting a ball is that when the individual is seated on the ball, her/his hips should be level with the knees. The firmness of the ball is another element to consider. A softer ball has a larger base or surface area, making it easier for the client to maintain balance. Firmer balls definitely provide more balance challenges. With specialized training, you can learn numerous exercises with stability balls. Because 80 percent of Americans suffer from a degree of low-back pain, the exercises shown with the stability ball have been chosen to strengthen the trunk musculature. Repeat all exercises 8 to 16 times.

Supine Trunk Curl

(Rectus abdominous, internal and external obliques)

Starting Position: Supine incline position with arms crossed over the chest or hands placed at the side of the head.

Action: Slowly curl your trunk, letting your shoulders and upper back lift off the ball. Return to starting position and repeat.

Tips: Support your head if your neck becomes fatigued. Think of bringing your ribs to your hips.

Variation: Change your feet position to vary the challenge of balance. The closer the feet are together, the more difficult it is to balance. Also, vary the position of your arms from across the chest, by the side of the head, or extended above the head.

Supine Oblique Rotation
(Rectus abdominous, internal and external obliques)

Starting position: Supine incline position with arms crossed over the chest or hands placed at the side of the head.

Action: Begin by bringing your ribs to the hips. As you curl your trunk, rotate one side of the upper body toward the other side. Return to starting position and repeat, rotating to the other side.

Tips: Always start each exercise with the trunk curl first. Press the lower back into the ball as you do the exercise.

Variation: Change your feet position to vary the challenge of balance. The closer the feet are together, the more difficult to balance. Also, vary the position of your arms from across the chest, by the side of the head, or extended to the f side of your torso.

Prone Trunk Extension
(Erector spinae, gluteus maximus)

Starting Position: Start prone with your trunk on the ball. Place your hands to the side of your head, by your side, or wrapped around the ball. Allow your trunk to round over the ball. Spread your legs and keep both feet solid on the floor.

Action: Slowly extend the spine, lifting your chest slightly off the ball until the spine is straight. Return to starting position and repeat.

Tips: Keep your neck in a neutral position. Do not overextend your spine.

Variation: Regularly change your arms from by your side, next to your head, or extended over your head.

Side-Lying Lateral Flexion
(Internal and external obliques, erector spinae, quadratus lumborum)

Starting Position: Start in a side-lying position on the ball with the bent leg firmly planted on the floor. Place one hand on the ball and bend the arm on the ball, placing the hand on the side of the head. Allow the trunk to round over the ball.

Action: Laterally lift the trunk slowly. Once you reach the top of the motion, return slowly to the starting position and repeat.

Tips: Do not allow your hips to roll forward or backward. Keep your head in its neutral position, not allowing it to dip down, forward, or backward.

Variation: As you get stronger, put both hands to the side of the head with your elbows to the side.

Stretch Right!

A well-designed flexibility program focuses on all the muscle groups and joints of the body—not just the most frequently used body parts. Stretch properly to achieve maximum flexibility.

Stretching Tips

- ❑ Stretch warm muscles, not cold ones.
- ❑ Avoid bouncing (ballistic) movement. Stretch gradually into and out of the stretch.
- ❑ Stretch to the point of limitation, not to the point of pain.
- ❑ Concentrate on relaxing the muscles being stretched; slow breathing helps.
- ❑ Stretches to improve flexibility should be held 15 to 30 seconds.
- ❑ Always stretch opposing muscle groups.
- ❑ Keep the muscles warm when stretching by wearing warm-ups or sweats.
- ❑ Stretch daily and certainly after every workout.
- ❑ Increases in flexibility take time; you must be patient.

Neck

Action: Very slow circular movement of head toward each shoulder and chest.

Tips: It is not recommended to take your head back too far—you may possibly stress your neck.

Shoulders (Two stretches)

1. Action: Holding a towel or rope over your head, stretch the arms back.

2. Action: Sit on the knees with the front of the feet flat on the floor. With towel behind back, bring the chest to the knees as you stretch the arms away from the body.

Tips: This is also a very good stretch for the spine and the front of the lower leg!

Variation: Change the width of your grip on the towel.

Hips, Side, and Back

Action: While sitting, bring one leg over other leg. Keep the bottom leg extended (but relaxed at the knee). Rotate the torso to both sides by pushing against floor with hands.

Tips: Look behind you and think "tall."

Lower Back

Action: While lying on the back, grab behind the knees and pull legs toward chest. May be done with legs tucked or slightly extended, but not locked.

Tips: This also stretches the hamstrings.

Variation: This stretch can be performed in the seated position.

Abdominals and Chest

Action: From a prone position, lift the shoulders and chest off the ground and support the upper torso with elbows or extended arms.

Tips: Reach up and out with the upper body.

Seated Butterfly Stretch
(For inner thigh)

Action: Bring both heels together and into body. Press knees toward the floor.

Tips: Grab your ankles, not your toes. Stretch torso forward as well.

Half-Straddle Stretch
(For hamstrings and lower back)

Action: With one leg straight and the other leg bent, reach your chest forward toward the straight leg and hold. Do both legs.

Tips: Keep the back straight and relax.

Straddle Stretch
(For hamstrings, inner thigh, and lower back)

Action: Stretch forward with your upper body between your open legs.

Tips: Keep your knees facing up, legs straight, and back straight. (Placing your hands on the floor behind your thighs is a good modification for those a little less flexible in this position.)

Quadriceps and Hip Flexors

Action: While lying on your side, grab below the knee and stretch the leg back.

Tips: Focus on bringing the leg back and not out to the side.

Variation: Do the stretch standing against a wall, next to a chair, or in the prone position.

Achilles Stretch and Calf-Stretch

Action: Stand in a lunge position with toes facing forward. To stretch the calf, bend front leg and keep back leg straight. To stretch Achilles tendon (and soleus), bend the back knee, keeping the heel on the floor.

Tips: Sometimes it is best to do these against the wall or an immovable object.

Yoga for Mind, Body, and Spirit

Though its exact origin in India has yet to be identified, yoga has existed for at least 5,000 years. Translated, yoga means union and refers to one of the classic systems of Hindu philosophy that strives to bring together and develop the body, mind, and spirit. Hindu priests who lived frugal lifestyles, characterized by discipline and meditation, originally developed yoga. Through observing and mimicking the movement and patterns of animals, priests hoped to achieve the same balance with nature that animals seemed to possess. This aspect of yoga, known as Hatha yoga, is the form with which Westerners are most familiar and is defined by a series of exercises in physical posture and breathing patterns. Besides balance with nature, ancient Indian philosophers recognized health benefits of yoga, including proper organ functioning and whole well-being. These health benefits have also been acknowledged in the modern-day United States, with millions of individuals regularly participating in yoga.

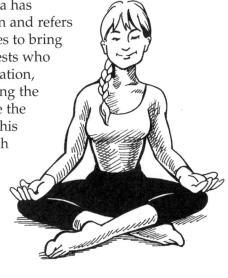

There are several different forms of Hatha yoga that are popularly practiced. Iyenhgar yoga incorporates traditional Hatha techniques into fluid and dancelike sequences. It uses props such as chairs, pillows, blankets, and belts to accommodate persons with special needs. Ashtanga yoga is a fast-paced, athletic style that is the foundation for the various power-yoga classes. These classes resemble more vigorous workouts as opposed to relaxation sessions. Bikram, or hot yoga, is done in a sauna-style room that's over 100 degrees, so the muscles get very warm for extending and stretching. Jivamukti is both physically challenging and decidedly meditative. Kripalu yoga centers on personal growth and self-improvement. Although each type of yoga will have its unique benefits, documented benefits from participation in yoga include the following:

- ❏ Increase in flexibility

- ❏ Increase in muscular endurance

- ❏ Increase in balance

- ❏ Improvement in posture

- ❏ Increase in caloric expenditure

- ❏ Increase in self-worth and self-control

- ❏ Reduction of stress

Section 5

Contemporary
Health Issues

Striving to be the healthiest person you can be is a very important goal in life. Your pursuit of optimal health emphasizes positive lifestyle practices and prevention strategies. Good health is determined by many of the choices you make in life about exercise, nutrition, weight management, alcohol use, smoking, substance use or abuse, and relationships. Developing your mind and managing your emotions are also closely interrelated with attaining optimal well-being. It is important that you take self-responsibility by engaging in activities that can positively affect your health. You deserve the opportunities that accompany good health. The purpose of this section is to briefly address some meaningful issues to help you make appropriate decisions regarding your personal health and well-being.

Self-Concept

Self-concept is how one feels about oneself. It is meaningful to note that someone with a low self-concept is more likely to adopt an unhealthy behavior such as smoking, alcohol, or substance abuse. A person's self-worth should come from the strength of his/her internal resources. Oftentimes an individual lets outside factors such as work, sports, school, or relationships determine his/her self-worth. This is very risky because these factors may be destructive to your self-concept. You need to acknowledge, to yourself, that you have positive attributes as well as faults, and that these qualities should not affect the decisions you make regarding your health. Clarify those physical, emotional, mental, and spiritual needs that must be met for you to be happy. Try to establish a link between your health behaviors and the fulfillment of these needs. This will help provide the direction and motivation for you to realize and sustain positive health outcomes.

The Balanced Eating Plan

Include a variety of wholesome foods in your total dietary intake. "Wholesome food" refers to food consumed in its natural state (or as close to its natural state as possible and free of additives, preservatives, or artificial ingredients) such as baked potatoes versus potato chips, raw fruits and vegetables instead of cooked and canned varieties, and whole-grain breads and cereals as compared to refined products. Processing often removes important nutrients. The best way to obtain the most vitamins and minerals is to eat food in its natural form.

Components of a Well-Balanced Diet

The balanced diet contains adequate amounts of carbohydrates, protein, fats, vitamins, minerals, and water.

Carbohydrates

Carbohydrates are the primary and most easily utilized source of energy your body. Did you know? Approximately 58 percent of your total caloric intake should come from carbohydrates. Refined and simple sugars, starches (complex carbohydrates), and fiber (cellulose) are the three forms in which carbohydrates are found in your food products. Refined sugars should be limited to approximately 10 percent of your daily carbohydrate intake. Complex carbohydrates, in the form of starches and naturally occurring simple sugars, should comprise the 48 percent balance of caloric intake from the carbohydrate food group. These are readily found in whole-grain breads, vegetables, and fruit. Your body uses carbohydrates, in the form of glycogen and glucose, to provide the energy for moderate, prolonged, and intense exercise and to contribute to the maintenance and functioning of your nervous system. In addition, under normal conditions, carbohydrates are the only energy source for your brain.

Proteins

Proteins are important for the healthy building and repair of every cell of your body. The essential amino acids, which cannot be manufactured within your body, must come from dietary sources. Americans tend to consume about twice as much protein as they actually need. Among key points to remember regarding protein are the following:

1. Proteins are important in helping to maintain your body's water balance.

2. Proteins in the blood help keep the acid level of the blood within a normal range.

3. Proteins are essential for you to have an immune response. This response produces antibodies to foreign substances that get into your system.

4. Many of your hormones are either protein or have protein components.

5. All of the many enzymes of your body are proteins.

6. Proteins act as carriers for a number of substances in your body.

7. Proteins play a role of passing information across spaces between nerves and muscles.

Did You Know?

Twelve percent of caloric intake should come from protein sources containing the essential amino acids.

Fats

You need some dietary fat and cholesterol to provide insulation, for energy, for the production of hormones, for absorption of certain vitamins, and as a vital component of cell membranes. The biggest dietary challenge for most Americans is to reduce fat consumption. Did you know? Total dietary calories from fat sources should be no more than 30 percent of daily food intake. Fats come in three important dietary forms: saturated, monounsaturated, and polyunsaturated. Saturated fats are found in animal products, including meats, poultry, and dairy products such as milk and cheeses. Tropical oils such as palm oil are predominantly saturated fat and are found in many prepared products. Saturated fat intake should be limited to less than 10 percent of daily caloric intake. The monounsaturated fats such as olive oil and polyunsaturated fats such as sunflower oil should comprise 10 percent each of daily caloric intake.

Unfortunately, elevated blood levels of fat have been linked to diseases of the cardiovascular system and to some forms of cancer. The typical American diet contains 43 percent of calories from fat. The process of reducing this level is difficult and probably more likely to be successfully changed when done slowly. However, the results in potentially better health are well worth the effort invested.

Water

Water is your most vital nutrient. More than 70 percent of lean body mass is water, whereas only 10 percent of body fat is water. Thus, lean body mass is mostly water, and fat is mostly fat. Water is an important constituent of all body cells. It surrounds the cells, permeates bone tissue, and is the foundation element of the circulatory system. Among its important functions are transportation of nutrients, removal of the by-products of cell metabolism, temperature regulation, joint lubrication, and cell structure shape. In addition, water is a medium for life-sustaining chemical reactions in the body. Drink an average of 8 to 10 eight-ounce glasses of water a day.

Vitamins

A well-balanced diet does not have to be supplemented to meet the daily vitamin requirements. However, a deficiency of one or more vitamins will result in some kind of symptom or deficiency reaction, whereas too much of a vitamin may cause a toxic reaction. Vitamins are grouped into two groups based on their solubility. There are the water-soluble vitamins (B vitamins and C) and the fat-soluble vitamins (A, D, E, K). Toxicity is more likely to occur with fat-soluble than with water-soluble vitamins. The best way to get vitamins in your body is from the foods you eat. Avoid low-nutrient foods like soft drinks and foods high in calories and fat. Nutrient-dense foods like whole grains and fresh fruits and vegetables will provide adequate daily caloric intake, as well as vitamins and other micronutrients. Beliefs that extra amounts of certain vitamins will give extra energy, reduce stress, prevent a variety of ailments, or improve endurance have not been proven by controlled research.

Minerals

The minerals, or micronutrients, are inorganic substances that your body needs in small amounts each day. They facilitate numerous functions in your bodily processes such as enzymatic activities, electrolyte balance, and fluid transport. They also have structural roles in the body.

Following are some general eating guidelines to help you design your all-around best-balanced eating plan.

Diet Guidelines

Meat and Protein Foods

- ❑ Eat less red meat; reduce the serving size and frequency.

- ❑ Eat fewer processed and cured meats (like ham, bacon, sausage, frankfurters, and luncheon meats high in saturated fats, sodium, and artificial preservatives).

- ❑ Select lean cuts such as eye round, sirloin tips, shoulder, chuck, flank, tenderloin, and remove all visible fat before preparing.

- ❑ Eat poultry (white meat without the skin), which has less saturated fat and fewer calories than beef or pork.

- ❑ Eat fish, which is low in fat. However, tuna, salmon, and sardines canned in oil contain more fat and less protein, so purchase them canned in water.

- ❑ Nuts and seeds are rich sources of vegetable protein but also contain a high concentration of calories and fat (mainly the "good" polyunsaturated kind). Sunflower seeds, sesame seeds, walnuts, almonds, and peanuts are the best sources.

- ❑ Although eggs are an excellent source of high-quality protein, the yolks contain a concentrated source of fat and cholesterol. Limit intake to three or four eggs a week, or eat only the whites of the egg.

Dairy Products

- ❑ Eat reduced- or nonfat dairy products such as skimmed milk, low-fat cottage cheese, plain yogurt, and low-fat cheeses. Reduce the amount of cream, ice cream (ice milk has about half the fat of ice cream), whole milk, whipped cream, and cream cheese. These products contain excess fat and calories.

Fats and Oils

- ❑ Use more polyunsaturated vegetable oils such as safflower, corn, and sunflower.

- ❑ Margarines high in polyunsaturates (usually the softer kind) are preferred.

- ❑ Avoid hydrogenated fats (the process that makes fats more saturated).

- ❑ Avoid palm oil and coconut oil, which are also high in saturated fat.

Fruits and Vegetables

❑ Eat raw fruits and vegetables daily. Many vitamins and minerals are destroyed in the cooking process.

❑ Eat dried peas and beans, which in their natural state are excellent lowfat sources of protein.

Breads and Cereals

❑ Eat whole grain breads and cereals, rather than refined ones. During the refining process, essential "B" vitamins and minerals are removed along with the bran (the outer layer of wheat kernel). Vitamin E is also lost when the wheat germ is expelled. Enriched breads and cereals replace many (but not all) of the lost nutrients.

Healthy Eating Tips

❑ Avoid eating large meals. A large meal elevates blood sugars and fatty acids. This extra food will usually be stored as fat in your body. Eat small meals at more frequent intervals throughout the day.

❑ Foods that are cooked, stored in the refrigerator (or freezer), and then reheated later lose many of their vitamins.

❑ Eat more slowly and chew your food completely. Fast eating encourages overeating.

❑ Avoid overusing the salt shaker.

❑ Limit consumption of cookies, cakes, and candies; they contain excessive amounts of sugar and fat.

❑ Read the label panels of foods to evaluate the nutrient content and look for hidden ingredients.

❑ Include more fiber in your diet. The typical American diet is too high in calories, sugars, fats, and sodium.

❑ Drink no more than two cups of coffee a day to avoid symptoms of anxiety such as nervousness, irritability, increased blood pressure, muscle tension, and difficulty sleeping.

❑ Avoid skipping meals (especially breakfast). Many times when meals are skipped, people more than make up for it at another meal.

❑ Spread your toast and bread with fruit-only jams instead of sugary jellies and butter.

❑ Satisfy your sweet tooth with low-fat treats such as frozen juice bars, nonfat yogurt, fresh fruit, and angel food cake.

❑ Toss your salad with gourmet vinegar and herbs instead of regular dressing.

- Eat air-popped popcorn at movies or for a snack.

- When buying peanut butter, choose the natural-style and pour the oil off the top.

- Use nonfat milk instead of cream or nondairy creamers in coffee.

- Give yourself permission to eat moderate amounts of the foods you enjoy on a regular basis.

- Get plenty of fiber. It is associated with lowered risk for cancer, diabetes, and coronary artery disease. Increase the amount of oats, beans, lentils, fruits, and vegetable skins.

- Add peanut butter and peanuts to your diet. Although there are fats in peanut butter, they are mostly monounsaturated while also being high in folic acid, thiamin, vitamin E, niacin, magnesium, zinc, and protein.

The Chocolate Fallacies

Everyone is entitled to enjoy eating chocolate in moderate amounts. However, some manufacturers would like to convince you that eating chocolate is more for health than pleasure. Here are some chocolate fallacies.

Fallacy #1: Eating chocolate doesn't make you fat.

In reality, no one single food does cause obesity. However, chocolate is a food with a lot of calories, so it is important to watch how much you eat for agreeable weight control.

Fallacy #2: Chocolate protects the heart.

It is true that one of the saturated fats in chocolate, called stearic acid, doesn't raise cholesterol. But chocolate has other saturated fats, such as palmitic acid, that do raise cholesterol. Also, it is meaningful to mention that stearic acid may help to promote blood clots, which can trigger heart attacks and strokes.

Fallacy #3: Chocolate helps to prevent cancer.

Chocolate does contain a high level of antioxidants, which are protective molecules for some cellular functions. Presently, many studies show the link between fruits and vegetables and a lowered cancer risk, but the studies on chocolate and cancer risk reduction are not here yet.

Bottom Line

For many of us, chocolate is a sweet sensation that is an utter enchantment for our culinary desires. In moderation, it certainly provides great fulfillment, with few harmful effects. It may be a wonderful delight, but at this time no research suggests it is a wonder food.

Food Guide Pyramid

The following pyramid illustrates the U.S. Department of Agriculture's recommended daily diet to ensure good nutrition and a variety of foods. It's not a strict prescription, but a general guide that lets you choose a healthful diet that's right for you. You will notice that it advocates using fats, oils, and sweets very sparingly. Also note that the new pyramid encourages greater consumption of fruits, grains, and vegetables.

Fats, Oils, & Sweets
USE SPARINGLY

KEY
▫ Fat (naturally occurring and added)   ☑ Sugars (added)
These symbols show fat and added sugars in foods.

Milk, Yogurt, & Cheese Group
2-3 SERVINGS

Meat, Poultry, Fish, Dry Beans, Eggs, & Nuts Group
2-3 SERVINGS

Vegetable Group
3-5 SERVINGS

Fruit Group
2-4 SERVINGS

Bread, Cereal, Rice, & Pasta Group
6-11 SERVINGS

Source: U.S. Department of Agriculture/U.S. Department of Health and Human Services

Reading Food Labels

Most foods in the grocery store must now have a nutrition label and ingredient list. Reading the new food label will help you choose healthy foods for your diet. Here are what some key words now mean on product labels as defined by the government.

Fat Free	Less than 0.5 gram of fat per serving
Low Fat	3 grams of fat (or less) per serving
Lean	Less than 10 grams of fat, 4 grams of saturated fat and 95 milligrams of cholesterol per serving
Light (Lite)	One-third less calories or no more than one-half the fat of the higher-calorie, higher-fat version; or no more than one-half the sodium of the higher-sodium version
Cholesterol Free	Less than 2 milligrams of cholesterol and 2 grams (or less) of saturated fat per serving

Note: g = grams (about 28 g = 1 ounce)
mg = milligrams (1,000 mg = 1g)

Make sure you check to see if your serving is the same size as the one on the label. If you eat double the serving listed, you need to double the nutrient and calorie values. If you eat one-half the serving size, cut the nutrient and calorie values in half.

Let the Daily Value be your guide. Daily values are listed for people who eat 2,000 or 2,500 calories each day. If you eat more, your personal daily value may be higher than what's listed on the label. If you eat less, your personal daily value may be lower. For fat, saturated fat, cholesterol, and sodium, choose foods with a low % Daily Value. For total carbohydrate, dietary fiber, vitamin, and minerals, your Daily Value goal is to reach 100 percent of each.

Nutrition Facts

Serving Size ½ cup (114g)
Servings per container 4

Amount Per Serving

Calories 90	Calories from Fat 30

	% Daily Value*
Total Fat 3g	5%
Saturated Fat 0g	0%
Cholesterol 0mg	0%
Sodium 300mg	13%
Total Carbohydrate 13mg	4%
Dietary Fiber 3g	12%
Sugars 3g	
Protein 3g	

Vitamin A	80%	Vitamin C	60%
Calcium	4%	Iron	4%

* Percent Daily Values are based on a 2,000 calorie diet. Your daily values may be higher or lower depending on your calorie needs:

		Calories	2,000	2,500
Total Fat	Less than		65g	80g
Sat Fat	Less than		20g	25g
Cholesterol	Less than		300mg	300mg
Sodium	Less than		2,400mg	2,400g
Total Carbohydrate			300g	375g
Fiber			25g	30g

Calories per gram
Fat 9   •   Carbohydrate 4   •   Protein 4

More nutrients may be listed on some labels.

Weight Management

Americans are battling with their weight. Investigations also show that 90 percent of dieters will regain the weight lost within a year or two, leading many people to just start a new diet. Although early conclusions from animal studies indicated that this yo-yo dieting (or weight cycling) was risky to your health, recent research from the National Institutes of Health now states that there is no conclusive evidence that yo-yo dieting is harmful to your physical health. A review of 43 human studies verify that yo-yo dieting does not lower metabolic rate, increase body fat, raise blood pressure, make it harder to lose weight the next time, or increase the risk of dying from heart disease. However, the emotional trauma from this weight cycling may be considerable.

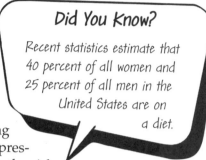

Did You Know?

Recent statistics estimate that 40 percent of all women and 25 percent of all men in the United States are on a diet.

Many weight-loss programs have directed their weight management interventions toward one single proposed cause of obesity. However, for long-term weight management, integrating several interventions will attain the best success.

Factors Influencing Obesity

Obesity may be defined as the percentage of body fat equal to or greater than 25 percent for men and 32 percent for women. It is associated with increased risk of cardiovascular disease, hypertension, diabetes, gallbladder disease, and certain cancers. According to an independent report of the Surgeon General on Health and Nutrition, the causes of obesity are poorly known, and therefore, education about how to treat this condition is lacking. Obesity appears to be influenced by

1. decreased physical activity,

2. high-fat diets,

3. genetics and,

4. behavioral factors.

A better understanding of these factors may help you design a favorable weight-loss plan.

Physical Activity

Did You Know?

According to the U.S. Department of Health and Human Services, only 22 percent of Americans engage in leisure-time physical activity at the level recommended for health benefits.

Physical activity has changed dramatically as our nation has evolved from an agricultural to industrial to technological society. Clearly 24 percent of adult Americans are completely sedentary, and the remaining 54 percent are inadequately active. This decline of physical activity has resulted in a significant decrease in daily caloric expenditure for the majority of Americans.

High-Fat Diets

Diet composition is now high in fat and refined sugar and low in starches and fiber. It is well documented that humans gain weight on high-fat diets. As a matter of fact, dietary fat is converted to body fat with approximately 25 percent greater efficiency than carbohydrates. Factors affecting this increased fat intake are expert retailers' pushing foods high in fat and sugar, fast-food restaurants, vending machines, and the fact that Americans are eating out more often.

The Genetic Factor

There is now conclusive evidence that body weight is considerably affected by genetics. The distribution of body fat in the body, principally in either the upper or lower body, is an inherited trait. Extra fat in the torso is associated more with men and increased health risk, whereas overfatness in the hips is associated more with women. If both parents are obese, it's very likely their offspring will also be overweight. Although the trend to develop obesity may be inherited, regular physical activity combined with a low-fat diet will definitely limit this genetic tendency if maintained throughout the life cycle.

Your resting metabolic rate is also a distinctive bodily process influenced by genetics. The resting metabolic rate (the energy required to maintain vital bodily functions including respiration, heart rate, and blood pressure) accounts for 60 to 75 percent of your daily energy expenditure. It may vary considerably between persons. For instance, the resting metabolic rate may differ by as much as 1,000 calories a day in obese women of the same height, weight, and age. In addition, investigations have shown that individuals with low metabolic rates gain more weight than persons with normal resting metabolic rates. The resting metabolic rate of women is about 5 to 10 percent lower than males because of less muscle mass. You can increase your resting metabolic rate with an increase in muscle mass through resistance exercise.

Did You Know?

The average percentage of fats in the American diet is about 43 percent, although the recommended percentage is 30 percent or less.

Fat cell number is another genetic factor that influences obesity. The average person has 25 to 35 billion fat cells in the body. Some obese individuals have up to three times the normal fat cell number. An individual experiencing continual weight gain may also produce more fat cells during adulthood. Unfortunately, once new fat cells have developed, a loss of fat will only result in a decrease in size but not number, leaving the individual with a higher number of fat cells. Mildly obese or overfat individuals usually have normal fat cell number. Weight gain in this case is associated with an increase in size and weight of fat cells.

Behavioral Factors

A number of the pioneer studies investigating the caloric intake of obese to nonobese subjects have revealed no appreciable difference in caloric intake between the two groups. However, new studies using technologically superior techniques for measuring caloric intake have shown that obese subjects typically underestimate their caloric intake by 30 to 35 percent. In fact, modern hospital- and university-based weight management investigations report binge eating disorders in 25 to 45 percent of obese individuals. Studies also show a strong link between psychological stress and binge eating. The implication of these results supports the importance of learning healthy eating habits as well as keeping accurate food inventories for persons in a weight-management program.

High-Protein, Low-Carbohydrate Diets: Debating the Diet Wars

Information technology is bombarding us with confusing and conflicting reports on what is the best way to achieve permanent weight loss. Some of the most popular diets now being touted are the high-protein, low-carbohydrate diets, which are in direct opposition to the recommendations of the majority of health, nutrition, and fitness professionals. Leaders in the high-protein, low-carbohydrate diets include Dr. Atkins's New Diet Revolution, The Zone, Protein Power, and the Carbohydrate Addict's Diet. Dr. Atkins asserts that cutting carbohydrates is the key to weight loss, because carbohydrates elevate your insulin levels, and insulin is a fat-producing hormone, converting blood sugar to stored fat. This statement is physiologically correct. The rise in insulin is the body's way of sending the blood sugar (glucose) to the brain and muscles for energy, with unused glucose being stored as fat. Dr. Atkins continues that by limiting the intake of carbohydrates, you avoid the rapid rise in blood sugar, which means less sugar will be stored as fat.

Other respected scholars argue that weight gain is more a function of consuming extra calories, regardless of the type of food (fat, carbohydrate, protein). They state that many people, when advised to eat more carbohydrates and less fat, take that as a message to eat as many carbohydrates as they desire. This "ticket to eat" inference has led many people into just eating more calories than they are expending, thus ensuring unwanted weight gain.

So why do people lose weight on these high-protein, low-carbohydrate diets? Some health professionals argue that the reason for the rapid weight loss in the high-protein, low-carbohydrate diets is attributable to a striking loss of water weight. This occurs for two reasons:

1. The body stores 3 parts of water to 1 part of carbohydrate. Significantly reducing carbohydrates will dramatically lower your water (not fat) weight.

2. By eating more proteins, the body's protein metabolism is enhanced, which requires the use of extra water for elimination of its byproducts.

Some researchers suggest that people are essentially just eating fewer calories on these high-protein, low-carbohydrate diet plans. Another possibility is that eating extra protein actually helps to curb your appetite, assisting you to eat less.

The high-protein, low-carbohydrate diets also claim that the body will more readily break down fat for energy over carbohydrates. This hypothesis hasn't been validated in studies, however.

Researchers have also studied high-carbohydrate, low-fat, and very low-fat diet regimes. These vegan-style diets have been very successful for people striving to lose weight. It is important to note that the carbohydrate selections include much more vegetables, fruits, grains, brown rice and beans, as opposed to French fries, cakes, and soda. They also promote fat-free yogurt and skim milk or their soy versions.

What about people who are insulin resistant? In the United States, approximately 10 to 25 percent of the population suffers from insulin resistance. These individuals are more susceptible to heart disease due to elevated blood fats, high blood pressure, and lower HDL (helpful) cholesterol. When insulin-resistant people consume carbohydrates, their insulin levels go up, but the body has difficulty utilizing the sugar for energy. Therefore some "experts" suggest these individuals should just eat fewer carbohydrates. However, reducing body weight and increasing physical activity are much more preferable ways to treat people with insulin resistance. Research has clearly shown that aerobic exercise and resistance training are very effective in improving one's sensitivity to insulin. Exercise promotes an efficient uptake of glucose for fuel. So, what should you do?

Although people can lose weight on the high-protein, low-carbohydrate diets, they may have grim health consequences. Let's face it, there is an abundance of research that suggests that depriving yourself of fruits and vegetables will increase your risk of heart disease, stroke, and cancer. It is well established that fruits and vegetables provide essential fiber and nutrients for healthy living. Also, because the water in your body constitutes anywhere from 50 to 60 percent of your weight, restricting carbohydrates may lead to dehydration. In addition, for any vigorous exercise regime, your body prefers carbohydrates as the primary fuel.

Perhaps, the best diet is one that does not wipe out carbohydrates, fats, and animal foods and is based on good old-fashioned serving sizes—eating in moderation. This may not result in the fastest loss of weight, but it is an attainable lifestyle for many that will in the long run lower your risk to coronary artery disease, diabetes, stroke, and some forms of cancer.

Fat Burner Supplements Flame Your Health Risk

You've all seen these promising ads about the revolutionary new fat burner supplements that burn off fat, even while you sleep. Their marketing has been quite effective, noting the success of a variety of fat burners you can purchase. They all contain one main ingredient: ephedra. Ephedra is a nervous and cardiovascular system stimulant. When used in a properly prescribed dosage, ephedra and its derivatives are effective in nasal decongestants. This herb will speed up numerous bodily processes, such as metabolism, heart rate, respiration rate, and blood pressure. Unfortunately, these bodily function increases may lead to harmful side reactions, including irregular heartbeats, chest pain, tremors, seizures, and other dangerous bodily effects.

Fat burner supplements are readily available at supermarkets, drugstores, and the Internet and range in price from $40 to $80 for a month's supply. Regrettably, the Food and Drug Association has little control over their sales and distribution. Drugs have to be researched and tested for safety before going on the market. Fat burners are sold as dietary supplements, which do not have to undergo the same careful scientific scrutiny as drugs. In addition, without federal regulation, the ephedra content varies greatly in different fat burner supplements, enhancing the impending risk. Several health and medical organizations are trying to warn potential users of the harmful side effects. Regardless, if you are aspiring to attain a supersculpted abdominal look or go down a dress size, achieve these bodily goals with a sound exercise plan and a healthy diet, not something that puts your life at risk.

Ten Strategies for Weight-Loss Success

Americans spend an estimated $35 million a year trying to lose weight. It's no secret that diet books, diet pills, packaged foods, liquid diets, weight-loss groups, and hospital-sponsored programs abound, and yet at this junction in time no single program, plan, or treatment offers long-term effectiveness to large numbers of individuals. A winning weight-loss program will not be as concerned with loss of weight as it is with loss of body fat. Follow these tips for weight-loss success.

1. **Don't go on a crash diet or fast.** Very low calorie diets, often referred to as crash diets, lead to quick loss of muscle and fat. Only a small number of dieters will reach their goal weight, and fewer than 5 percent will maintain their new weight. Fasting exposes the body to a condition that actually increases the activity of fat-depositing enzymes. Your body is reacting to what it perceives as starvation conditions and tries to protect itself from not being supplied the necessary foodstuffs.

2. **Go for fat loss—calories count!** The best diet to promote fat loss is a well-balanced, low-fat, heart-healthy, high-carbohydrate eating plan composed of a variety of foods to ensure good nutrition. It is important to educate yourself on which foods are high in fat and which are low. A rule of thumb for caloric expenditure is to consume roughly 16 calories per pound for moderately active people and no less than 1,200 calories a day. A high-carbohydrate, low-fat diet is also recommended for lowering the risk of high blood cholesterol, coronary artery disease, and high blood pressure.

3. **Exercise works.** The exercise program is essential to the success of any weight management plan and should be composed of aerobic exercise and resistance training. A powerful benefit of aerobic exercise is that it enables the body to more efficiently burn calories and use fat for fuel. Resistance training will gradually increase muscle mass, increasing the body's basal metabolic rate. Therefore, you will be burning more calories at rest, too.

4. **Food choices.** Choose food that is low in calories but high in nutrients. Eat more complex carbohydrates such as whole-grain breads, cereals, rice, vegetables, bran products, and oatmeal. Substitute sugar-rich desserts with fruits. Drink plenty of water. It is a major component of your body and provides the environment within which the other nutrients may function. Eat low-calorie, nutrient-dense foods for snacks to help control your hunger between meals. Watch your consumption of alcohol. Alcohol has plenty of calories, but no nutrient value. Limit your salt intake to that which occurs naturally in food.

5. **Weight-loss goals.** Establish safe weight-loss goals. A loss of up to two pounds per week is a healthy recommendation for weight loss. Avoid seeking that slender fashion model figure. This may be too unrealistic and could lead to psychological distress and diet failure.

6. **Eating habits.** Many people eat till they are too full, mainly because the food tastes so good. Take responsibility and use good judgment at your meals. Also, it is not healthy just to eat when you are hungry. Instead of two or three large meals a day, eat five or six smaller ones, which better distributes your caloric needs throughout the day. Eat at a slower pace to avoid overeating and stomach discomfort.

7. **Food doesn't solve problems.** Unfortunately, conditions such as stress, emotional distress, or loneliness may lead some individuals to use food as a way of dealing with the problem. Attempt to disassociate food with these issues and seek professional counseling if necessary to establish appropriate intervention strategies. Food is an enjoyable fuel for life, not a mood-heightening support system.

8. **Behavior modification.** A major goal of any successful weight management program is to modify behaviors that may contribute to the problem. Begin by identifying those factors that may reinforce behaviors that are counterproductive to your body fat goals. Two helpful behavior modification measures involve the application of knowledge and values. Knowledge of accurate nutrition and exercise information is invaluable to complete your successful plan. Establishing new values enables you to develop behaviors that improve your quality of life and attain your body fat goals. Maintaining a positive attitude will certainly help.

9. **How to choose a good diet.** Choosing a safe and effective diet may be difficult with the hundreds of "miracle" diets on the market. Avoid programs that advertise unique fat-burning enzymes or fat-reducing formulas, as no known formulas exist. Stay away from the quick and easy promises—there is no fast and easy way to lose excess fat. Steer away from those one-food diets, as they are deficient in essential nutrients. The program should be low in calories but complete in essential nutrients. It should incorporate a variety of food choices that you enjoy. Make sure the diet fits into your way of life. It should be designed to reduce no more than two pounds of fat per week. Finally, the diet you select should have lasting potential. Ask yourself if you can maintain it for a lifetime.

10. **Lifetime changes.** The dietary, exercise, and behavior changes you make should be sustainable for a lifetime. Develop a faithfulness and appreciation for exercise and health, not an obsession with thinness.

Substance Abuse

Alcohol

As reported in *Healthy People 2000*, the costs of alcohol problems in America were estimated to exceed $70 billion per year, with the majority of these costs attributed to reduced productivity. It is second to tobacco as the leading cause of premature death.

> ### Did You Know?
> Alcohol is indicated in nearly half of all deaths caused by motor vehicle crashes and fatal intentional injuries such as homicides and suicides.

Some general reasons people drink alcohol:

❑ It often serves as a medium for friendship when people meet "for a drink."

❑ It is frequently used to celebrate an event.

❑ It is a means of dealing with stress, anxiety, emotions, or depression.

❑ It is commonly used in social situations to lessen fears and make people feel at ease.

❑ It is a lure successfully used by clever advertisers.

❑ It is a behavior often introduced by role methods.

Alcohol Continuum

Researchers have identified an alcohol continuum from which people may be able to evaluate or assess themselves or others.

- ❑ An *occasional drinker* drinks in small amounts, usually on special occasions.

- ❑ A *light drinker* drinks regularly in quantities that are not intoxicating.

- ❑ A *social drinker* drinks moderately, but in quantities that are not intoxicating.

- ❑ The *problem drinker* drinks to the point of intoxication, following no specific pattern or even realizing what is happening.

- ❑ The *binge drinker* drinks heavily. Usually the drinking is linked to issues arising at work, home, or within his/her social life.

- ❑ The *chronic alcoholic* has problems associated with long-term, uncontrolled, and frequent drinking.

| Does Not Drink | Occasional Drinker | Light Drinker | Social Drinker | Problem Drinker | Binge Drinker | Chronic Alcoholic |

Women and Drinking

A variety of unique problems may arise when women drink. Females tend to have more body fat than men, and alcohol concentrations tend to be higher in people with more body fat. With less muscle mass than men and less water in their tissues (fat tissue has very little water), alcohol is absorbed into the bloodstream faster, even when all other absorption variables are constant. Therefore, a man and woman with the same body weight, who have consumed the same amount of alcohol in the same time period, will find the woman to be more intoxicated (primarily due to her body fat content). The effects to the fetus of a mother who drinks are well documented. Fetal alcohol syndrome is the second-highest cause of mental retardation in the United States. This is entirely preventable!

Drink Responsibly

The amount of alcohol in a person's bloodstream at a given time is referred to as one's blood alcohol concentration (BAC). The liver metabolizes 0.5 ounce of alcohol per hour. This is equivalent to the following drinks: 12 ounces of beer, 12 ounces of a wine cooler, 5 ounces of wine, or 1.5 ounces of liquor. It takes approximately one hour for any of these drinks to be metabolized by the liver and the BAC to return to normal. If more alcohol is consumed than is metabolized, the BAC will rise, and signs of impairment in motor skills, speech, equilibrium, and decision making will increase accordingly.

It is your responsibility to keep your BAC low and your behavior under control. Be aware of the reasons you may be drinking and make responsible decisions of how much you drink, what you drink, your limitations, your attitudes toward others who drink, and the consequences associated with alcohol use.

Tobacco

One out of every six deaths may be attributed to smoking. The use of tobacco is closely linked to diseases of the cardiovascular system, a number of cancers, respiratory infections, and ulcers.

The active ingredients in smoking tobacco are nicotine, tar, and carbon monoxide. Nicotine, which is extremely addictive, stimulates the production of epinephrine. This causes the blood pressure and heart rate to increase and blood vessels to constrict. Tar, similar to that on city streets, is a sticky fluid that settles in the lungs and inhibits their functioning. Carbon monoxide is a deadly gas that retards the effective transportation of oxygen through the bloodstream.

> **Did You Know?**
>
> According to the Surgeon General, smoking is the single most important preventable cause of death in the United States.

The rate of female smokers is on the upswing whereas it is decreasing for the rest of the population. This increase in women smokers has been attributed to a desire of some females to have a slender image. This same desire makes it very difficult to quit smoking, as there usually is a small gain in weight that accompanies smoking cessation. The important point to stress is that smoking is a far greater risk to a person than gaining a few extra pounds.

Tobacco is consumed in five different forms:

1. cigarettes
2. low-tar and nicotine cigarettes
3. clove cigarettes
4. cigars and pipes
5. smokeless tobacco

Although the low-tar and nicotine cigarettes are proposed to be safer, many of these smokers actually increase their cigarette consumption to satisfy their need for tar and nicotine. Smokeless tobacco (snuff or chewing tobacco) use is increasing, especially among young males. It is not a safe alternative for people who wish to quit smoking. Cancer of the cheek and gums is 50 times higher among smokeless tobacco users.

To quit smoking is a difficult process that requires breaking both a psychological and physical addiction to nicotine. It is very difficult for smokers to quit on their own. There are several programs available that utilize a number of approaches (behavioral, psychological, sociological, and pharmacological) that have proven to be successful in helping people stop smoking. With the cessation of smoking, a number of positive improvements in health rapidly occur. These include:

❑ improvement in sense of smell and taste,

❑ more efficient food digestion,

❑ better circulatory and cardiorespiratory function,

❑ better heart efficiency,

❑ improvement in breathing capacity.

Other Drugs

Drug use can be found throughout every area of the country, in all social levels, at all income levels, and within many group affiliations. It is associated with a number of health problems including overdoses, drug-related violence, injuries, HIV infection (from shared needles), and birth defects. Oftentimes the use of drugs begins with harmless curiosity and results in substance abuse and dependence. Signals of drug dependence include the following:

1. emotional withdrawal,

2. decline in academic performance,

3. loss of interest in usual activities,

4. change in social groups

5. concern with obtaining money, and

6. cranky behavior.

There are several categories of substance abuse drugs, which include the following.

❑ **Psychedelics.** The psychedelics or hallucinogenic drugs produce sensory and perceptual distortions of reality that may be pleasant or terrifying. Many of these drug episodes will last up to 12 hours and cannot be ended early.

❑ **Opiates.** Heroin, long a part of the drug world, has similar but more powerful pain-relieving properties than morphine. Its main ingredient is opium, which is very addictive.

❑ **Central nervous depressants.** Barbiturates are central nervous system depressants that may depress muscle control, speech, anxiety, and mood.

❑ **Central nervous stimulants.** Cocaine and amphetamines are central nervous system stimulants. Amphetamines are occasionally used to curb appetite and to cope with difficult situations, such as cramming for tests. Babies of women who are cocaine users during pregnancy are more likely to have birth defects. Stimulant drugs often result in behavioral disturbances, irritability, hostility, and unprovoked violence. It should be noted that caffeine and nicotine are also central nervous system stimulants.

- **Marijuana.** Marijuana is probably the most used illegal drug in the country. Attempts have been made to legalize it, with activists proclaiming marijuana less dangerous than tobacco or alcohol. However, the smoke in marijuana is harmful to the respiratory system. Although the long-term use of marijuana is unknown, chronic use of marijuana has been associated with infant mortality and neurological problems.

- **Deliriants.** Designer drugs fall into this class. These are illegal drugs intended to replace some of the various street drugs.

A variety of programs are accessible to help people break their drug habits. Many treatment programs use substitution drug therapy. Counseling and support groups are also available. The most desirable solution to drug abuse is prevention. There are numerous ways to enjoy the gratification of a healthy life without having to depend on the dangerous stimulation of drugs.

Stress Maintenance

Stress is an inevitable part of living. Life does have its ups and downs. Excessive stress and burnout can have emotional consequences.

One of the main causes of stress is a sudden, drastic, unwanted change: personal loss in the family, a job crisis, injury or illness, financial problems, and emotional problems all fall into this category. The tension from stress often leads to that worried, uptight sensation we call anxiety—you feel angered or frustrated. If these feelings continue to obstruct your ability to enjoy life, physical ailments such as ulcers and high blood pressure may result.

Being "stressed-out" may even lead to depression. Do you recognize the symptons of depression?

- restlessness

- feelings of inadequacy and insecurity

- inability to concentrate

- sleeplessness

- lack of interest in food, life, and social interaction

You can beat it! You can take charge!

Follow these guidelines:

1. Talk over your problems with a close friend or seek professional advice. You need to express your feelings!

2. See a physician if you have any physical ailments.

3. Do vigorous exercise regularly to vent anxiety and to combat depression.

4. Don't overload yourself. Set practical goals you can reach successfully and timetables you can meet.

5. Learn to relax. You need some peace and quiet each day just for **you!**

6. Organize your work and personal affairs. This will give you more efficient use of your time and will rid your life of clutter.

7. Take short breaks or a vacation. Time out will give you a better perspective.

8. Look ahead. Sometimes you can anticipate a job slump, a budding problem, or financial difficulties and be prepared.

9. Stay away from drugs and alcohol—they are just temporary relievers of tension, not cures for problems.

10. Improve your eating habits and your diet. Don't skip meals because you are too busy.

Stress Release Breathing Intervention

Here's a simple breathing drill you can do anytime to help lesson the effects of stress. Sit very comfortably and focus on relaxing your muscles in your body, especially those that are tensing up. Keep your breathing very slow and controlled. As you inhale say to yourself, "I am," and as you exhale say to yourself, "relaxed." Continue for 3 to 5 minutes.

Technology to Technostress

Although the benefits of technology are enormous, a new, unexpected type of stress is technostress. Technostress is the anxious feeling one gets by feeling reliant on technological devices (computers, fax machines, voice mail, remote control devices, pagers, etc.). Thanks to technology, more people than ever before are adopting sedentary lifestyles, while spending hours at a time on a computer.

What Are Some Symptoms of Technostress?

A common symptom is diminished concentration. People feel as though their memory is failing them, forget what they started to do, misspeak words, can't find the right words, or lose their train of thought. Impatience and irritability are also other symptoms. When you are technostressed it is difficult to find time to relax.

So, What Are Some Technostress Busters?

One simple suggestion is to go outside for a walk. Just being in the outdoors, in nature, appears to be most beneficial. Start an outdoor hobby such as gardening, hiking, or biking. All types of exercise are beneficial including aerobic exercise, resistance training, and flexibility training.

Avoiding Burnout

Everyone has the potential to suffer from burnout. The end result is a diminished capacity to function efficiently. Oftentimes the high demands needed for success, criticisms from others, and unrealistic expectations are underlying themes to burnout.

How to Avoid Burnout

1. Be careful of working long hours; in the long run this can lead to fatigue and loss of motivation.

2. Overextending yourself: try not to solve all of the world's problems. Get involved but be discriminate about your capabilities.

3. Too much stress, frustration, and anxiety in your situation may lead to burnout.

Signs of Burnout

1. Attitude shift toward negativity; you may start putting less effort in current projects or an indifference towards your work.

2. Exhaustion; look for signs of frequent illnesses, fatigue, or even sadness.

3. Feelings of inadequacy; you may feel moody and less competent in areas in which you are really more talented, educated, and skilled.

Some Ways to Reduce Burnout

1. Be a good listener to your body. If you are regularly ill, exhausted, and fatigued, your body is warning you that something is wrong.

2. Realize you cannot do everything and be realistic on what you can accomplish.

3. Examine your work hours and perhaps incorporate some time-management practices.

4. Don't overbook yourself.

5. Learn something new. Sometimes the boredom of work can take its toll. Go to some guest lectures or a seminar on a topic of interest. Pick up a new book to read.

6. Do something different. Perhaps you might find much satisfaction in having a pet or starting some type of hobby. Be willing to try something you've always considered, but never felt you had the time to do.

7. Do something different in your job. If possible try to do something different in your job that breaks you from the mode you might be experiencing. For instance, teachers might start using multimedia in the classroom to bring more visuals to the lectures. Students might want to buy some new video learning aids now available in most college bookstores.

Finally, try to draw a line in your life from who you are and what you do. Allow time for some of your friendships to grow and reestablish your lifestyle values for home and happiness.

The Seven Energy Bolsters

Do you ever get that feeling you want more energy? Do you know what to do? Here are some simple but effective tips you can do to bolster your energy.

1. Start by eating healthy and enough. Oftentimes the restrictive diets people attempt lead to early fatigue and low energy. Also, these same diets are often deficient in important vitamins and minerals your body needs to stay healthy.

2. Drink more water. A good rule of thumb is to drink about 1/2 to 1 cup of water every hour you are awake.

3. Get your carbohydrates. Without a doubt, carbohydrates are the most influential nutrients that regulate your energy. Eat plenty of whole-grain breads and cereals, rice, potatoes, pasta, and beans.

4. Take your vitamins and minerals. You may wish to consider a multivitamin if you know your daily diet seems insufficient. Key energy vitamins to focus on are vitamin C, calcium, magnesium, and potassium.

5. Keep an eye on iron. It is no secret that iron deficiency is a prevalent cause of fatigue in women. Don't forget that tofu and kidney beans are good sources as well as lean red meat.

6. Don't skip breakfast. Breakfast will help maintain your blood sugar levels.

7. Sleep on. It is important to get the adequate sleep your body needs. Losing only one or two hours can sometimes sap you in the day.

8. Exercise. Aerobic exercise and resistance training improve several metabolic processes that can all lead to increased energy.

Creative Problem-Solving

Whether it's solving a school issue, a personal challenge, or a family dilemma, resolving a problem can be quite stressful. When faced with this type of task, use these 10 ways to help resolve your predicament.

1. **Clearly define the problem.**

2. **Explore all possible solutions.**

3. **Be positive** and optimistic that you are going to successfully resolve this issue.

4. **Discuss and analyze** this problem and possible solutions with others who you respect. Choose colleagues who show a sincere interest in your well-being.

5. **Don't be overly critical** of any resolution ideas.

6. Allow yourself to **be imaginative** during this process.

7. Sometimes a new or different solution makes you feel apprehensive. **Feel confident** that it is O.K., because you are using a fresh problem-solving approach.

8. **Summarize your options.**

9. **Choose a resolution** direction and put it into action.

10. **Observe and evaluate.** If the problem is not resolving, you may need to try another one of your options.

Creative problem-solving is quite challenging. Reward yourself (with a book, show, or something special to you) for having gone through this process, as this method demands powerful analytical thinking and problem-solving skills.

Time Management Tips

Let's face it, time management for everyone can sometimes get pretty outlandish. With personal responsibilities, family responsibilities, work responsibilities, school responsibilities, and much more to do, it is no wonder many people find themselves overloaded. Use these eight tips to help you anticipate, organize, and take charge of your time.

1. **Start a master schedule.** Write down all your goals, commitments, and things to do. Make sure this master schedule is updated daily. This is also a good time to evaluate whether you have taken on too many projects and need to "put something on hold" for a later date.

2. **Organize and prioritize** your goals and commitments. Now that you have a master schedule, prioritize everything to keep you on track. Allow this organizational process to be very fluid, as goals and objectives often shift in importance.

3. **Focus on the big picture.** It is easy to lose a lot of energy micromanaging things that are of less importance. Focus your attention on what needs to be accomplished, in the order you have established.

4. **Be wary of regular distractions.** Telephones, pagers, mobile phones, fax machines, and e-mail can become distractions to accomplishing tasks. Sometimes it is best to allocate priority work times when you will not accept incoming communications and other possible distractions.

5. **Project breakdown.** Many people find it more productive and efficient to break down a large task into miniprojects.

6. **Establish a realistic time line for projects.** This may be the most difficult step. However, by creating a realistic time line you are helping yourself to avoid procrastination.

7. **Be an "objective detective" time manager.** An objective detective time manager can regularly anticipate the unexpected, such as more time needed for an assignment, and readjust his/her master schedule accordingly.

8. **Block into your life some daily "flex time."** Try to have some time each day that is allocated flex time to take care of projects that need more time or for you to get ahead on other coursework.

Be a Great Communicator

Life is a constant state of communication with friends, colleagues, employers, teachers, and others. Here are eight instructions to improve your professional and personal relations by being a more effective communicator.

1. Look at the other person. Always **make eye contact** with the person you are communicating with in a live conversation. This reflects self-confidence on your part.

2. **Listen actively** to the other party. Focus on the conversation without thinking of other things.

3. **Stay on track.** Some discussions start to digress when one or both parties begin to bring up unrelated issues or pointless past events.

4. **Avoid being judgmental.** Always try to be objective and comprehend the other person's point of view.

5. **Be sensitive and respectful.** In all conversations and discussions, appropriate respect and sensitivity to the feelings of others is appreciated.

6. **Clarify and then repeat.** Try not to assume anything in a conversation. Clarify important points and repeat statements to verify that what you heard was correct.

7. **Observe body language.** Oftentimes others may project their feelings with their body language. Observe the hands, face, and posture, and note how this person is expressing himself or herself nonverbally.

8. **Be supportive and constructive.** In all conversations make a point to be constructive and supportive in your feedback.

Section 6

Fitness Facts and Fiction

Frequently Asked Questions

General Health

1. **What are three major factors that contribute to improved health?** Regular aerobic exercise, improved dietary habits, and a positive mental attitude.

2. **Will exercise make you tired?** Only temporarily; exercise will ultimately give you more energy.

3. **Will exercise enhance your sex life?** You bet! Increased energy, more vitality, higher self-esteem, stress control, and body firmness all contribute to a person's sex life. Right?

4. **Will exercise give you a longer life?** The aging process cannot be reversed, but exercise may slow down normal physiological deterioration. More importantly, exercise can improve the quality of your life.

5. **What qualities do people who have lived to be 100 have in common?** Moderation and a positive outlook on life. Few smoke and few are fat. They usually get up early and go to bed early. Many claim to have always kept busy during their lives and describe themselves as hard workers. They all seem to be very self-sufficient and protect themselves from too much stress.

6. **How does smoking affect exercise?** Smoking constricts the bronchial tubes, which are the pathways by which oxygen and other gases enter the body. Also, the carbon monoxide in cigarette smoke can combine with hemoglobin in red blood cells, taking space that should be used to transport oxygen to the exercising muscles. Thus, your cardiorespiratory system must work harder to do the same amount of work.

7. **Can exercise really improve your mental health?** Yes, studies have shown that exercise brings about both short- and long-term psychological enhancement and mental well-being. Some of the psychological benefits from physical activity include improvement in self-confidence, relief of tension and feelings of depression, positive changes in mood, increased alertness, clearer thinking, and positive coping strategies. Individuals of all ages and gender can realize these benefits from exercise.

8. **Does the distribution of body fat have any health consequences?** Yes, people who gain fat in the abdominal area have a higher risk of coronary heart disease, high blood pressure, diabetes, and stroke as compared to individuals who gain fat in the hip area. Men tend to gain fat around the waist and women at the hip.

9. **Why do people who exercise have fewer colds and viral infections?** It has been observed that exercise may boost the immune system and that physically active people take better care of themselves. It should be noted that regular, strenuous exercise has also been shown to have an opposite effect on the body's immune system. This adds support for an exercise prescription directed toward regular, moderate levels of exercise participation.

10. **I read a lot about the health benefits of soy. Are they true?** Soy has been shown to be very health beneficial. For instance, research shows that soy consumption will lower triglycerides and LDL-cholesterol (lousy cholesterol) in people with high blood lipids, while raising the HDL cholesterol (helpful cholesterol). Note also that heart disease is much lower in Asian countries, where soy is a dietary staple. Soy also has been shown to play a role in lowering breast and uterus cancer.

11. **How does soy improve one's health?** It is felt that the hormone phytoestrogen mimics some of the effects of estrogen, actually blocking off some of the harmful effects associated with estrogen. Also, remember that soy foods are low in saturated fat and are cholesterol free. For an Internet source on soy-based foods and products, go to www.soyfoods.com.

12. **As you age, is there anything you can do to slow the decline in mental process?** The degree of decline varies from person to person, but the age-related changes are due to alterations in the brain's frontal lobe, right behind the forehead. However, new research suggests that sedentary older people who take up aerobic exercise (such as walking) can slow the loss in mental ability even if they never exercised before in their lives. Researchers believe that the aerobic activity improves mental functioning by increasing the supply of oxygen to the brain.

13. **I have trouble sleeping. Do you have any suggestions to get a better night's rest?** Try to establish a sleeping schedule of going to bed the same time every night and getting up at the same time each morning. Work on the stress levels in your life, as this can dramatically affect sleep. You sleep better if the room temperature is slightly cooler than other parts of the house. Try to avoid drinking too many fluids before bedtime so that your bladder isn't full. Remember, spicy foods for dinner, or as snacks, may cause heartburn or stomach acidity and impair your quality of sleep. Also, avoid alcohol near bedtime. Although it may help you fall asleep, when the alcohol wears off your brain actually becomes more alert. Finally, stay away from sleeping pills, as they may lead to unwanted side effects and health-related risks.

14. **I use a computer everyday. Are there any exercises that will help prevent and control carpal tunnel syndrome?** Carpal tunnel syndrome is a condition that develops from repetitive wrist motions such as typing at a computer terminal. This motion may lead to pressure on the median nerve in the wrist and great pain and discomfort. Do the following exercises throughout the day. Frequently take your wrists through a complete range of motion in both directions. Make a tight fist with both hands, hold for 6 seconds, and repeat 3 to 4 times. Also, circle your wrists in both directions while holding your hands in a fist. Make sure you take short breaks from your typing to do these exercises (and to rest your wrists) to safeguard from developing carpal tunnel syndrome.

15. **What is hypoglycemia?** Hypoglycemia means low blood sugar. Most individuals may be affected by what is referred to as reactive hypoglycemia, a condition resulting from glucose levels dropping after a meal or when you haven't eaten for several hours. Symptoms include dizziness, anxiety, shaking, and uneasiness. Eating small, but frequent meals and avoiding concentrated sources of sugar is recommended.

16. **Can you tell me in minutes or days how much smoking reduces life?** According to some research, every cigarette a man smokes reduces his life by 11 minutes. Each carton of cigarettes represents a day and a half of lost life. For every year a man smokes a pack a day, he shortens his life by about two months.

17. **What's the latest on St. John's wort?** St. Johns wort is a very popular "feel-good" herbal supplement. Many people take it to fight depression and lift their spirits. The scientific evidence is quite convincing that it is effective for treating *mild* depression for a short period of time, around two months.

    Alas, there is no evidence that it will elevate your mood if you are not mildly depressed, so don't rush out to buy it in hopes of making you feel more cheery. Most studies with St. John's wort have lasted no longer than 6 weeks, so the long-term benefits are really unknown.

    Lastly, St. John's wort may lessen the effect of certain medications, so always speak to your physician or a pharmacist before taking this herbal supplement.

18. **What should you look for when buying a new pair of sunglasses?** Sunglasses shield your eyes from dust, wind, ultraviolet (UV) rays, and glare. Look for the Z80.3 sticker that ensures the shades protect against all types of ultraviolet light. Sunglasses labeled "cosmetic use" and "general purpose" usually offer less protection. Surprisingly, the tint has nothing to do with the protection; it's the chemical coating in the lens that blocks the UV rays. However, brown, gray, and green are pretty much the best colors for general-purpose vision because they don't distort colors. For skiing, boating, and sports where light is reflected, you probably need special-purpose sunglasses, which block UV and a lot of visible light. The plastic and polycarbonate lenses are better at blocking UV rays then untreated glass. Plus, they are impact-resistant. Although comfort and style will always be important in your choice, try to select sunglasses that don't block your peripheral vision; safety should always prevail over outward show.

19. **How are colds and flu viruses spread?** Cold and flu viruses are usually spread by shaking hands with the infected person or by touching something the infected person recently held. You will infect yourself by then touching your mouth, eyes, or nose. To prevent exposure, wash your hands regularly when around people with colds and flu viruses. Also, coughing and sneezing can transmit viruses, so keep your distance from those who are ill.

20. **What's the most common joint injury people have in the United States?** According to the American Academy of Orthopaedic Surgeons, ankle sprains are the most common joint injuries. Your ankles are regularly transmitting forces equal to three to four times your body weight when you run and jump. Up to 85 percent of the ankle injuries are inversion sprains. This is when the sole of the foot turns inward, injuring the ligaments on the outside of the ankle. As with any joint injury, the symptoms are pain, tenderness, and swelling. Remember, treatment for sprains is R.I.C.E: Rest, Ice, Compression, and Elevation.

21. **Is there any merit to these hair analysis ads to detect nutritional deficiencies?** Don't be wowed by these ads. Your hair is predominantly a protein called keratin, plus some small amounts of fat and melanin, which gives your hair its color. Hair analysis cannot detect nutritional deficiencies or detect any diseases for that matter. Your hair does not contain any vitamins, and the mineral levels are not realistic values to measure for any health assessment.

22. **Is second-hand smoke dangerous?** Yes, second-hand smoke has been shown to be associated with increased risk of heart disease, lung and breast cancer, and breathing-related diseases.

23. **Does cold weather give you colds?** People exposed to chilling temperatures often feel they are more susceptible to colds. However, it is viruses that give you colds, not the weather. Colds are actually more common in cold weather because people are inside more, and thus more exposed to germs.

24. **How do you avoid repetitive strain injuries?** With the wonderful benefits of computer use, there are also some physical perils to know. Repetitive strain injury (RSI) results from hand, wrist, arm, and neck injuries from a repetitive (fast) work. Carpal tunnel syndrome is a form of RSI that results from pain in the tendons and nerves across the wrist. To avoid, take frequent breaks during your typing and make sure your computer set up avoids any neck, back, wrist, and eye strain (see *Sitting at Your Computer Station* on page 41).

25. **Are the sunless tanning lotions safe?** According to the U.S. Food and Drug Administration they are safe. The main ingredient in self-tanning products is dihydroxyacetone, which reacts with the top layer of skin to form a light brown tan stain. Remember that these lotions do not give you any sun protection, however.

26. **How successful are all the stop smoking interventions?** The interventions range from acupuncture, nicotine gum and patches, hypnotism, antidepressants, and behavior modification approaches. None of the methods has outstanding long-term effects, with each method showing a 20 percent success rate after one year. Quitting smoking is essential. A person needs the support of the family and friends as well as a sustained effort to find the intervention that works.

27. **What causes your limbs to "fall asleep"?** A limb will become numb when you remain seated or lying in a position that compresses a nerve in the limb or stops the blood flow to the nerve. This sometimes happens when you cross your legs or arms for an extended period of time. When you remove the pressure, the tingling is the nerve sensitivity returning. Moving the limb helps to speed up the recovery. Men who carry a thick wallet in their back pocket (with tight pants) can put pressure on the sciatic nerve, causing a similar numbness and pain.

Exercise

28. **Should you exercise on hot, humid days?** Keep it light. Sweat will not evaporate well (to cool you off) in the humidity, and you may overheat.

29. **Are those so-called "sports drinks" beneficial during exercise?** The composition of these drinks is basically water, electrolytes (minerals capable of carrying an electrical charge), and glucose. Sweat consists mostly of water and electrolytes. In prolonged endurance events, glucose (carbohydrate) replacement may be beneficial. Also, endurance exercise in heat contributes to heavy losses of water and electrolytes, which need to be replenished.

30. **Is it O.K. to drink water while exercising?** Yes, your body's circulation system must get food and nutrients to the working cells to carry out their chemical reactions. Sweating during exercise depletes your body's water supply, which may lead to dehydration. Do not depend on your thirst to tell you to drink water. Try to drink at least 8 ounces of cool water for every 30 minutes of vigorous exercise. Use that water bottle!

31. **Should additional salt be taken after exercise?** There's plenty of salt from the food we eat and what we sprinkle on it. Excess salt can irritate the stomach, dry out body tissue, and raise blood pressure.

32. **Will I get more out of my workout by speeding up the exercises?** No, smooth, controlled movements, properly executed through the full range of motion at an even tempo, are more important than speed.

33. **Do all exercise programs give the same benefits?** No, but everyone needs sustained, full-body, moderately paced aerobic activity.

34. **What training effects happen to your body with aerobic exercise?** (1) Your lungs will be able to process more oxygen. (2) The heart becomes a stronger muscle and pumps out more blood with each beat (stroke volume), which in turn allows you to increase oxygen delivery. (3) The blood vessels offer less resistance to blood flow, reducing the work of the heart. (4) The working muscles become more efficient at utilizing oxygen and nutrients for energy (ATP).

35. **How long does it take to realize the benefits of a regular exercise program?** It takes about four to 12 weeks for benefits to appear and up to six months for you to get "hooked" on exercise.

36. **How many days of exercise can you miss before beginning to lose what you've gained?** No more than three days in a row.

37. **How long can you completely lay off exercise before you lose it all?** From five to eight weeks.

38. **What is muscle soreness and how do you get rid of it?** There are actually two types of muscle soreness: acute and delayed onset muscle soreness, or DOMS. Acute soreness occurs during or

immediately after a workout. It is hypothesized that this type of soreness is the result of the accumulation of metabolism by-products in the muscle. DOMS appears one to three days following the workout and lasts for up to two days. The latest research suggests DOMS is caused by microscopic tears to the connective tissue (surrounding the muscle fiber) and to some muscle fibers. Performing the same activity (at a lesser intensity) that caused the muscle soreness will help relieve it.

39. **What is that pain in the side sometimes felt in aerobics?** That sharp pain below the rib cage, often called a "stitch in the side," is usually caused by poor circulation in the muscles of the diaphragm or rib cage. Slow down your pace to allow the proper dilation of the affected blood capillaries, and the pain will go away.

40. **What is cross-training?** Cross-training is a method of integrating different fitness activities with the purpose of gaining or maintaining total-body fitness while reducing injuries. Each person must find the best mix of aerobics, resistance training, swimming, cycling, racquet sports, walking, and recreational sports. It is a very safe, effective, and balanced approach to fitness. Cross-training is extremely effective in a weight-loss program, as total work and hence caloric expenditure can be increased without increasing the risk of overuse injuries.

41. **Explain what steady state and lactate threshold mean?** Steady state in aerobic exercise represents a balance between the oxygen needs of the working muscles and their oxygen supply. As exercise intensity increases, the oxygen supply to the working muscles cannot meet all the oxygen needs of the muscles, and therefore, anaerobic energy systems will contribute more to the total energy production of the working muscles. The eventual transition of predominantly aerobic, oxidative energy production to include more anaerobic energy production during increasing exercise intensity is referred to as the lactate threshold, or onset of blood lactate.

42. **Why do you perspire more after you stop working out?** During exercise, your muscles need most of the blood to get oxygen for the activity. Upon the cessation of exercise, more blood is diverted to the skin to cool the body by means of sweat production. Also, during most modes of exercise, you are moving a lot, which helps sweat evaporate more efficiently during the activity.

43. **I only have time right before bed to exercise and am worried that it will impair my evening sleep patterns.** Interestingly enough, recent research has shown that vigorous exercise ending 30 minutes before bedtime failed to disrupt sleep.

44. **What causes muscle cramps?** New research on exercise-associated muscle cramping suggests the cramp occurs as a result of abnormal nerve activity from the spine, probably related to fatigue. Although not well understood, it is believed that tired muscles going through repeated shortening contractions are more vulnerable to cramping. Avoiding overfatiguing workouts and incorporate regular stretching to best ward off muscle cramps.

45. **What does the term "MET" mean?** This term is used to describe energy expenditure of an activity. One MET is equivalent to the energy expenditure of a person at rest. It is expressed in terms of oxygen uptake (i.e., 3.5 ml O_2/kg/min). It is very much like a shorthand method of describing energy requirements. For instance, running 6 miles per hour is about 10 METs, whereas walking 3 miles per hour is about 3.3 METs.

46. **What are the limiting factors of flexibility?** With the muscles relaxed, and reflex mechanisms minimally involved, researchers have found the relative contributions of soft tissue to joint stiffness to be the following: joint capsule, including ligaments (47%), muscles and their fascial sheaths (41%), tendons (10%), and the skin (2%).

Nutrition

47. **Do vitamins enhance performance and give energy?** A **surplus** of vitamins probably won't improve your performance. Vitamins don't contain energy, food does, but vitamins **do** help metabolize food.

48. **What is the difference between saturated and unsaturated fats?** Saturated fats come predominantly from animals and are a suspected contributor to coronary heart disease. Unsaturated fats come from vegetables and are much better for your system.

49. **What are the best foods to eat after aerobic exercise?** A selection of foods rich in complex carbohydrates (starches, not sugars), such as whole-grain breads and cereals, pastas, potatoes, leafy vegetables, green beans, broccoli, rice, peas, fruit, and grains. But give your body about an hour to recover first!

50. **What is dietary fiber?** It is basically a type of complex carbohydrate made up of plant material that cannot be digested by the human body. Refining and processing foods removes almost all of the natural fiber. The main sources of dietary fiber are whole-grain cereals and breads, fruits, and vegetables. Optimal amounts of fiber in the diet increase gastric motility and therefore may reduce the incidence of diverticulitis, colon and rectum cancer, and obesity.

51. **Is it O.K. to drink beer after working out?** Alcohol is a diuretic, which means that it stimulates urine production. Following a workout you want to replenish your body with lost fluids. Consequently, drinking any alcoholic beverage before or after exercise is not recommended.

52. **Are natural vitamins better for you than manufactured vitamins?** No, your body can't distinguish the difference between vitamins manufactured in a laboratory and natural vitamins extracted from food.

53. **What's a good substitute for those high-fat potato chip snacks?** Try pretzels. They are almost fat free. As a matter of fact, pretzels are one of the fastest-growing snack foods in the United States. However, there is good news for you chip lovers. There are now some new and improved chips that are low in sodium, fat, and calories. Read the labels at your supermarket. Look for the chips that are baked, not fried, and avoid chips made in hydrogenated oil. Remember to check the total fat content and serving size, too.

54. **Can you drink too much caffeine?** Most people have internal regulators that tell them when to stop drinking caffeine. However, 4 to 6 cups of coffee a day may result in symptoms referred to as caffeinism: breathlessness, headache, lightheadedness, and

irregular heartbeat. Too much caffeine may also trigger a panic attack. For college students, caffeine-containing soft drinks have overtaken coffee as the primary source of caffeine. Most experts advise no more than 200 milligrams of caffeine consumption, which is about the same as two to three 5-ounce cups of coffee.

55. **Are there any foods that will make you more satisfied and less likely to binge?** Yes, some of the most filling foods include boiled potatoes, steamed fish, oatmeal, oranges, apples, whole-wheat pasta, grilled lean beef, baked beans, grapes, and whole-grain bread.

56. **What is grazing?** Grazing is an eating plan some people have adopted where they eat frequent little meals (up to six) spaced throughout the day. For some people, this may help to control the appetite, and they actually consume fewer calories. The one downside of this eating plan is the time it takes to plan, prepare, and then eat the smaller meals.

57. **What is this creatine supplement craze?** Creatine is an amino found predominantly in the muscles in the form of creatine phosphate, where it facilitates energy production. It also helps to reduce the lactic accumulation during intense exercise. Most investigations have shown that creatine supplements boost short-term muscle strength and power. However, it is important to note that the long-term effects of high doses of creatine are unknown.

58. **Is it true that when you eat out, you usually eat more calories than at home?** Yes, large portion sizes and high-fat entrees burden most of this responsibility. Be aware that when you go out you are less likely to eat nutritious food. Forego eating appetizers, as they add to the calories. Perhaps split a dessert as opposed to ordering one for yourself. Also, most Americans neglect fruits and vegetables when eating out.

59. **What is the difference in brown rice versus white rice?** The nutty flavor and chewy texture of brown rice is due to it retaining the grain's bran. Brown rice has slightly more vitamin E, magnesium, and some other minerals. It also has more grams of fiber than white rice.

60. **I am so rushed to get things done that I am contemplating taking some of these liquid meal replacements on a regular basis.** Many of these liquid meals provide plenty of calories as well as a number of minerals and vitamins. But typically they do not provide the health promoting fiber and phytochemicals that are found in fruits and vegetables. So, this is not to discourage their consumption, but make sure you balance their intake with real meals.

61. **What does it mean when a food has the American Heart Association logo on it?** The red heart with white check mark means no more than 3 grams of fat, 20 milligrams of cholesterol, and 480 milligrams of sodium. The food must also have at least 10 percent of the daily value for one or more of these nutrients: protein, vitamin A, vitamin C, calcium, iron, or dietary fiber.

62. **What's the final scoop: Butter or Margarine?** Good question. Although margarine is indeed lower in saturated fat than butter, it's higher in trans fatty acids, which do contribute to high levels of cholesterol. Recent research does suggest that margarine is healthier. Also, it appears that soft tub margarine may be the best overall choice.

63. **What is the most common nutritional deficiency in the United States?** Iron deficiency. It affects some 8 million women of childbearing age and upwards of 700,000 toddlers.

64. **What is this new concept of training called periodization?** Although not really new, it is now being used regularly with recreational resistance-training enthusiasts. Periodization is most widely used in resistance training and involves systematically alternating high loads of training with decreased loading phases to improve components of muscular fitness. The system is typically divided into three cycles: (1) The microcycle, which lasts up to seven days; (2) The mesocycle, which can be from two weeks to a few months, is subdivided into preparation, competition, peaking, and transition phase; and (3) The macrocycle which is the overall yearly training period.

65. **What is carbo loading and how do you do it?** Carbo loading is a method of supersaturating your muscles with glycogen. It has been shown to improve endurance performance in events lasting over 90 minutes and is often used in competitive events. About seven days out from the event, begin by eating a diet high (60 to 70 percent) in high glycemic carbohydrates such as rice, pasta, and potatoes. Make sure you are getting adequate amounts of fat and protein as well. Drink plenty of water and increase your water intake four to eight cups (above normal) about two days before the event. Avoid dehydrating drinks and foods. As the event comes closer, remember to taper down your training so your body will be appropriately rested for the contest.

66. **What are phytochemicals?** They are not vitamins. They are not minerals. Phytochemicals are plant chemicals that offer great health benefits. They have been shown to protect against heart disease, cancer, diabetes, osteoporosis, and other medical conditions. The only way to get phytochemicals is to eat or drink them in fruits, vegetables, juices, nuts, and whole grain products.

67. **Can vegetarians get enough protein?** Yes, vegetarians who eat a wide variety of foods each day will absorb a full complement of essential amino acids (the protein building blocks your body can't synthesize). Nuts, seeds, legumes, and many grains are good sources of protein. Also, vegetarians don't need to eat the complementary proteins at the same meal.

68. **Is it true that tea may possibly be a healthful beverage?** Yes, black and green teas (sorry, not herbal teas) appear to lessen cholesterol's damaging affect on your arteries, as well as protect against cancers of the skin and gastrointestinal tract. Make sure you steep tea for 3 minutes for the beneficial antioxidants in the leaves to enter the beverage.

69. **I like juice with pulp. Does it have more fiber than juice without pulp?** There is no significant difference in the fiber between juice with pulp and juice without it.

70. **What are trans fatty acids and are they good or bad for you?** Trans fatty acids are unsaturated fats that have had hydrogen added to them, making them more saturated. This chemical process helps to extend the shelf life of many foods, such as crackers, cakes, cookies, chips and unsaturated oils (such as corn and soybean). Regrettably, trans fatty acids raise your total cholesterol and LDL or "lousy" cholesterol. They can also lower your helpful or HDL cholesterol. In addition, trans fats, as they are sometimes called, are associated with increased risk of diabetes. When looking at food labels, the words *partially hydrogenated* indicate there are trans fats in the food, but the label typically doesn't say

how much. Perhaps the best advice is to consume less processed and fast foods, as they have the most trans fatty acids.

Weight Management

71. **Can you reduce the number of fat cells in your body?** No, only the size of the fat cells, not their numbers.

72. **What is the fastest way to lose weight?** Weight management is a balance of energy intake (food) and energy output (exercise). The most efficient method for reducing "fat" weight is to do more aerobic exercise and resistance training and eat less food.

73. **Can you lose weight by diet alone?** Certainly, only you lose
a lot of muscle tissue as well as fat. You need exercise, too!

74. **What is the recommended percentage of fat for men and women?** From 5 to 15 percent for males 18 to 34 years of age, and from 16 to 28 percent for women 18 to 34 years old.

75. **How is the percentage of body fat determined?** Several popular methods include skinfold calipers, underwater weighing, and electrical impedance analysis.

76. **Is there a difference between being overfat and overweight?** Yes, overweight is only concerned with pounds. Overfat is concerned with the muscle/fat relationship. For instance, many professional football players are overweight by the familiar height/weight charts but have a low percentage of body fat (under 14 percent) and are certainly not overfat.

77. **What is your Basal Metabolic Rate (BMR)?** It is the minimal energy requirements of the body at rest. It can be simply estimated by multiplying your body weight in pounds by a factor of 10 or 11 for women and men, respectively. For example, the basal metabolic rate of a 120-pound female is (120 x 10) 1200 calories per 24 hours.

78. **What happens to your BMR as you age?** Your BMR decreases with age primarily for two reasons. (1) There is often a loss of lean body tissue (muscle) with aging. (2) There is usually a decrease in activity while diet remains constant. This is all the more reason to keep exercising throughout your life!

79. **In a typical group-exercise class consisting of 20 to 30 minutes of aerobic exercise, will loss of excess body fat be maximized at a lower or higher exercise intensity?** Although it is true that exercising at a lower intensity burns predominantly fat and at a higher intensity predominantly carbohydrates, at the higher intensity, total caloric expenditure of fat and carbohydrate will be greater. Therefore, a person should exercise at the highest exercise intensity that can be safely maintained for the exercise period if loss of excess body fat is the primary goal of the exercise program.

80. **Why does the mirror show your change of shape before the scale?** Muscle is denser than fat. A pound of fat bulges out 18% more than a pound of muscle. Because you are adding muscle to your body as you shape up, you will often notice a loss of inches before a loss of weight.

81. **Is yo-yo dieting risky for you?** Let's face it, many well-intentioned diets do fail, which has concerned researchers that the losing and regaining of weight might be harmful to the body. However, new research with high blood pressure, which is a major risk factor for heart disease, shows that yo-yo dieting doesn't appear to have any physiological damage. However, in terms of emotional wellness, yo-yo dieting may be most detrimental.

82. **Why don't diets work?** Most diets, especially fad diets, are poorly designed plans that unrealistically restrict caloric intake. You lose weight initially, but these plans are not permanent weight-loss eating strategies, which people can incorporate into a regular lifestyle. Consequently, individuals usually return to their previous eating habits that encouraged the weight gain in the first place. Eating habits (and exercise) must be changed permanently for diets to be successful.

83. **Will eating spicy foods help you burn more calories?** If you want to boost your metabolic rate, it's not going to be by eating spicy foods. Just because you feel hot and sweaty, it really has little to do with your metabolism. The best way to boost your metabolic rate is by doing regular resistance exercise.

Disease

84. **How do age and gender affect coronary heart disease risk?** Generally, the older you are, the greater your risk for heart attack. Between the ages of 35 and 44, coronary heart disease is less frequent in women than men, probably due to the production of the female hormone estrogen. Heart attacks appear to even out with older age.

85. **What are the four most important coronary heart disease risk factors?** Cigarette smoking, high blood pressure, abnormal levels of cholesterol, and physical inactivity.

86. **Is there any evidence that exercise can reduce heart disease?** Yes, a scientific study of over 16,000 Harvard alumni suggests that people who expend 2,000 calories per week in brisk exercise reduce death rates from heart disease by 25 to 33 percent, compared to those who do not exercise. Death rates decreased with increased weekly calorie expenditure up to 3,500 calories, after which there was no advantage to those who did more exercise.

87. **What are free radicals and antioxidants?** Free radicals are unstable molecules produced by chemical reactions utilizing oxygen in the body's cells. A variety of external factors can promote free radical formation including smoking, drinking alcohol, and pollution. Antioxidants (vitamin C, E, and beta carotene—a precursor to vitamin A) protect the cells from free radicals by neutralizing the process of molecular oxidation that leads to their formation.

88. **What are the leading causes of death in the United States?** According to the National Center for Health Statistics, they are heart disease, cancers, strokes, injuries, chronic lung diseases, pneumonia, diabetes, suicide, AIDS, and homicide.

89. **What is cholesterol?** Cholesterol is a fatlike substance used to help build cell membranes, make some hormones, synthesize vitamin D, and form bile secretions that aid in digestion. Because fat can't mix with water, which is the main ingredient of blood, cholesterol's most important job is to help carry fat through your blood vessels. Before cholesterol can enter the bloodstream it is coated with a protein, referred to as a lipoprotein. Lipoproteins are transport vehicles in the circulation plasma that are composed of various lipids such as cholesterol, phospholipids, triglycerides, and proteins known as apoproteins. The major classes of lipoproteins are chylomicrons, very low-density lipoprotein cholesterol, low-density lipoprotein cholesterol, and high-density lipoprotein cholesterol.

90. **Which is the "bad" and "good" cholesterol?** The low-density lipoprotein cholesterol (LDL-C) is the primary transport carrier of cholesterol in the circulation. It is referred to as the "bad" cholesterol because too much cholesterol, from eating foods high in saturated fat, often leads to LDL-C pieces adhering to the inner walls of the blood vessels, narrowing the blood passages. On the other hand, the high-density lipoprotein (or helpful) cholesterol's (HDL-C) primary function is to transport cholesterol from the tissues and blood to the liver for excretion or recycling. It is referred to as the good cholesterol.

91. **What are triglycerides?** Triglycerides (TG) are fats that circulate in the bloodstream that provide energy for the body. It is uncertain whether high TG levels are associated with coronary heart disease. However, high TG levels are associated with diabetes, kidney diseases, and obesity. Steps to lower TG levels include cutting down on saturated fat, losing weight, exercise, and quitting smoking.

92. **I've heard recent reports that eating an egg or more a day isn't that bad for your heart after all.** More controlled research is needed. The American Heart Association and U.S. Department of Agriculture suggest no more than 300 milligrams a day of cholesterol intake. One egg has 215 milligrams of cholesterol, which leaves you only 85 milligrams for any other foods.

93. **Will exercise reduce a woman's risk to breast cancer?** Exercise reduces the risk of heart disease, diabetes, stroke, and obesity. It appears to have a protective effect against breast cancer, but more research is needed. However, the best advice for men and women is that they should exercise.

94. **What dietary substances are needed to prevent osteoporosis besides calcium and vitamin D?** Two other substances of importance are magnesium and potassium, which are both found in fruits, vegetables, milk and whole grains.

95. **I read a recent study that said high-fiber diets don't cut colon cancer.** Even if the study was well-conducted research, it is still only one study. Decades of research suggest that high-fiber foods are a protection against colon cancer. Remember, stay away from those sugary sweets that are consistently associated with colorectal cancer.

96. **How can I, as a young man, protect against prostate cancer?** Very wise preventative measure. Prostate cancer is the second leading cause of cancer in American men. Research confirms that diets high in fat, calories, and animal products are strongly associated with this deadly disease. Diets high in grains, cereals, soybeans, nuts, and fish, on the other hand, appear to have protective effects.

97. **What are the most common types of arthritis?** There are actually more than 100 different forms. Osteoarthritis is a wearing and tearing form that affects the fingers and weight-bearing joints (knees, back, hips). Rheumatoid arthritis causes irritating joint stiffness and swelling. Fibromyalgia leads to pain at different points of the body as well as insomnia, morning stiffness, and constant fatigue. Gout is caused when uric acid accumulates in the joints, specifically the big toe, knees, and wrists. Lupus can damage the kidneys, heart, skin, lungs, and joints.

98. **What does "prediabetes" mean?** The American Diabetics Association and the U.S. Department of Health and Human Services now use the term prediabetes describe blood sugar levels that are higher than normal. Left untreated, many individuals will develop diabetes within 10 years. Losing 5 to 10 percent of body weight and doing at least 30 minutes of aerobic exercise daily will return blood sugar to normal.

99. **Is it true that eating big meals is associated with heart attacks?** Yes, a meal high in calories may quadruple the risk of a heart attack in those at risk to coronary heart disease. Researchers theorize that the large meals may temporarily elevate blood pressure, which could break loose some atherosclerotic plaque in an artery. This free-floating plaque in the bloodstream could lead to a blood clot in a coronary artery. Enjoy your meals, but eating in moderation is good for heart health as well as weight control.

100. **I thought all I had to be concerned with for heart disease is checking my cholesterol and triglyceride levels. What's this new protein associated with heart disease?** There's a new clue in understanding heart disease. It involves how the body's immune system works. The development of atherosclerotic plaque (hardening of the arteries) triggers the body to begin an inflammatory process to try to heal the artery wall. With some people, this inflammation process leads to ruptures of the atherosclerotic plaque. This could break off a piece of plaque into the bloodstream and be a precursor to heart attacks (if the clot goes to the heart) or a stroke (if the clot goes to the brain). The best blood predictor for this inflammation process, which is very easy and inexpensive to measure, is called hs-CRP for high sensitivity C-reactive protein.

　　If you have high levels of hs-CRP you can reduce the risk of heart disease by eating a diet low in saturated fat and cholesterol, lose weight if you are overweight, do regular aerobic exercise, stop smoking if you smoke, and control your blood pressure.

101. **What is heartburn?** Heartburn occurs when gastric fluids, which are very acidic to better digest food in the stomach, enter the esophagus. If this happens frequently, the esophagus may develop scar tissue and be more susceptible to developing cancer.

Sixteen Exercise Myths

1. **If you are thin, you're fit.** Sorry, but being thin is no indication of how efficient your heart, lungs, and muscles are. Body composition testing has demonstrated that many thin people actually have more than the recommended percentage of body fat. You've got to exercise!

2. **Sit-ups get rid of stomach fat.** Wouldn't that be nice! This myth is based on spot reducing. Research clearly shows that exercises for specific body areas firm the muscles, but fat reduction comes from aerobic exercise and a decrease in caloric intake. Fat is reduced proportionally throughout the body.

3. **Weight lifting develops aerobic capacity.** Lifting weights does elevate the heart rate, but this type of exercise does not improve aerobic capacity. It does develop firmer and shapelier bodies.

4. **Sweat loss means weight loss.** You do lose weight temporarily when you sweat, but this is mostly water loss, not fat loss, and is regained as you quench your thirst. Similarly, "sauna sweat suits" induce a temporary water loss and can be dangerous if you get too dehydrated.

5. **Aerobic exercise and jogging cause a woman's breasts to sag.** There is no evidence documenting this claim. However, a good supportive bra is recommended for comfort.

6. **Extra protein makes you stronger.** Wouldn't it be great if there really were superfoods? If you eat a well-balanced diet, you should consume enough protein for your body's needs. Excess protein is only converted into and stored as fat.

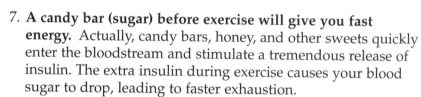

7. **A candy bar (sugar) before exercise will give you fast energy.** Actually, candy bars, honey, and other sweets quickly enter the bloodstream and stimulate a tremendous release of insulin. The extra insulin during exercise causes your blood sugar to drop, leading to faster exhaustion.

8. **Go for the burn.** Listen to your body. Any type of pain is a warning signal. None of the physiological mechanisms associated with "the burn" have been demonstrated to have beneficial results for you.

9. **Lifting weights gives women bulky muscles.** Women do not produce enough male hormones to allow for large muscle growth. And women don't have as much muscle fiber or mass as a man. Lifting weights will help a woman develop a better figure.

10. **A low resting heart rate means you're fit.**
Exercise can lower your resting heart rate.
However, this alone does not indicate a
person's fitness level.

11. **Electrical stimulation can
reduce fat, increase tone, and
build strength.** Wow, all those
results for just sitting there with
electrodes attached to you.
How appealing! Though
electrical stimulation devices
are used by physical therapists
for rehabilitation purposes, they
are quite ineffective as an
effortless exercise alternative.

12. **Muscles turn to fat when you stop exercising.** There are
many retired athletes who seem to prove this. However,
fat cannot change to muscle (or vice versa). When you
stop exercising, your muscles start to waste away and
lose their firmness. If you continue to eat a substantial
diet (as many of these athletes do), the overconsumption
of food will result in larger fat cells.

13. **Cellulite is a unique type of fat.**
Cellulite is fat; all fat is fat.
Sometimes excess fat bulges
between connective tissues under
thin skin giving that "cellulite"
appearance. Rubbing creams don't
work. Remove cellulite through
aerobic conditioning, body firming
exercises, and a proper diet.

14. **There is major physiological
deterioration as we age.** Although there is a slight
tendency toward reduced performance with age, in
general, people continuing their aerobic exercise maintain
much of their aerobic efficiency and exercise capacity.

15. **Free weights are better than machines.** Not so fast. There are advantages of both modes of resistance training.

  ❑ **Machines:** Machines ensure that you go through a standardized movement pattern, while targeting specific muscles. The newer exercise devices also have built-in safety features for the user. Several machine designs provide an effective variable resistance through the movement range to make exercises more challenging. Lastly, the exerciser doesn't have to balance the weight when training with machines.

  ❑ **Free Weights:** For many trainers, having to balance the weight, as is the case with free weights, is an advantage because this involves more stabilizing muscles. Free weights offer much more versatility in their use from the way you hold the weight, as well as your position using the weight. The inexpensive cost of free weights is a major advantage. Finally, free weights allow the user to go through different planes of motion than machines, which have fairly fixed planes of motion (although some companies have now developed this feature with some machines.)

16. **Weight gain is inevitable as you get older.** Actually, this is more related to a reduction in physical activity as opposed to age. With inactivity a person loses muscle mass, which reduces the metabolic rate at which they expend calories. At the same time, this inactivity leads to a gradual accumulation of body fat. The best way to prevent this is to include aerobic exercise and resistance training into your daily life.

Fitness Trivia Quiz

Try this trivia quiz to learn some additional fitness facts!

1. True or False: The average foot walks more than a thousand miles a year.

2. Is it training **affect** or training **effect?**

3. True or False: Muscles waste away if they are not used.

4. What percent of your body weight is water? 40%, 60%, 80%.

5. True or False: There are over 600 muscles in the human body.

6. What unique dynamic ability do muscles possess?

7. Which is the single most important source of fuel for your body? Fats, carbohydrates, proteins.

8. What is the junction of two bones called?

9. What is the term for enlargement of muscles?

10. True or False: It only takes 23 seconds for blood to circulate through your entire body.

11. One pound of fat equals how many calories?

12. The average heart beats how many times a minute? 62, 72, 82.

13. Name four of the six classifications of nutrients you need to eat.

14. True or False: Vitamins contain calories.

15. True or False: Vitamins are named as alphabet letters because, when they were discovered, scientists did not know their chemical structure and could not give them "proper" names.

16. Lack of what mineral is associated with "tired blood"?

17. True or False: Your appetite increases in cold weather.

18. Fast-twitch muscle fiber, known for its explosive characteristics, is referred to as _____ muscle fiber. (red or white)

19. What is the longest muscle in the body?

20. What is the largest tendon in your body?

21. Your skeleton comprises what percent of your body weight? 15%, 25%, 35%.

22. How many years does it take for the cell structure of your skeleton to completely rejuvenate itself? 5 years, 7 years, 10 years.

23. True or False: Two-thirds of exercise-induced injuries are caused by overuse.

24. Which is the only joint in the body with 360 degrees of rotation?

25. True or False: Sweat is your body's way of cooling off.

26. What is the single most preventable cause of death?

27. True or False: Women live approximately eight years longer than men.

28. True or False: Current estimates in the United States indicate that over 50 percent of all adults have a weight problem.

29. How many glasses of water should you drink each day?

30. True or False: Drinking cool water during exercise is beneficial because it reduces internal body heat.

Answers on page 151.

Health Trivia Quiz

Try this trivia quiz to learn some additional health facts.

1. What is the least favorite day of the workweek?

2. A specific fear associated with a place, thing or person is called a _____.

3. True or False: In the United States more women smoke than men.

4. True or False: Studies show that 85% of teenagers who occasionally smoke two to three cigarettes (a day) go on to become nicotine dependent.

5. Women can reduce infant mortality by _____% if they stopped smoking. 10%, 20%, 30%.

6. True or False: Drinking alcohol helps a person attain restful sleep.

7. True or False: Alcohol increases one's creativity.

8. If someone is addicted to alcohol, what is the best way to change this addiction?

9. True or False: Pathological gamblers are not intelligent people.

10. True or False: Shopaholics often make unnecessary purchases because the process of buying is often more important that what is bought.

11. True or False: Workaholics are driven perfectionists who would rather work than play.

12. True or False: If you consume a lot of protein you also need to increase your water intake.

13. True or False: Eating foods with fiber helps you manage your weight better.

14. True or False: If you eat too much sugar you will get diabetes.

15. Which is more nutritious: fruit juices or fruit drinks?

16. What constitutes a low-in-sodium food?

17. What is a processed food?

18. What neurotransmitter in the brain is associated with well-being and depression?

19. What cycle determines your body's blood pressure, temperature, hormone output, cell division, and sleep/wake cycles?

20. Is it better to try to go to bed at the same time nightly or wake up at the same time every morning?

21. What is the leading cause of nonfatal injuries in the United State and second-leading cause of death from injury?

22. What age group is prone to getting bored?

23. The causes of 90 percent of high blood pressure are uncertain and referred to as _____.

24. Heart attacks occur most frequently on what day?

25. The heart's built-in heartbeat comes from where?

26. Is heart disease reversible?

27. What type of tumor contains tissues not typically found where they originate?

28. What is it called when unwanted cells in the body spread like seeds to other parts of the body?

29. What is a fake solution or fake cure to a health problem called?

30. What is the single most important thing you can do to prevent the transmission of infectious organisms?

Answers on page 152.

Answers to Fitness Trivia Quiz

1. True
2. Training effect
3. True
4. 60%
5. True
6. They contract
7. Carbohydrates
8. A joint
9. Hypertrophy
10. True
11. 3500 calories
12. 72
13. Carbohydrates, fats, proteins, water, vitamins, minerals
14. False—vitamins do not contain calories
15. True
16. Iron
17. True
18. White
19. Sartorius on the thigh
20. Achilles tendon
21. 15%
22. 10 years
23. True
24. Shoulder
25. True
26. Cigarette smoking
27. True—One of the primary reasons for this is the higher incidence of heart attack deaths among men before the age of 55.
28. True
29. 8 to 10 eight-ounce glasses
30. True

How Did You Do?

26 or more correct   You are Exceptional!!!
21 to 25 correct   You can be Proud!!!
16 to 20 correct   You should Try Harder!!!
15 or less correct   You are Not Alone!!!

Answers to Health Trivia Quiz

1. Monday

2. Phobia

3. False—Actually, more men (31%) smoke than women (26%). However, women who do smoke are heavier smokers and usually start at younger ages.

4. True

5. 10%

6. False—Alcohol interferes with normal sleep rhythms.

7. Although drinking alcohol may reduce one's inhibitions, it does nothing to improve your productivity or creativity.

8. The majority of alcoholism practitioners agree that giving up drinking entirely is the best solution.

9. False—They often have superior intelligence.

10. True

11. True—Workaholics are obsessed with their career and making a living.

12. True—Protein requires seven times more water than carbohydrate and fat for metabolism.

13. True—Foods high in fiber are low in fat and have a bulking effect in your stomach that aids in the feeling of fullness.

14. False—Diabetes results from two problems: an increased insensitivity of the body's cells in the presence of insulin and an insufficient production of insulin by the pancreas.

15. Fruit juice, which will be low in sodium and high in potassium.

16. 140 mg of sodium or less per serving

17. Food that has been cooked, mixed with additives, or altered in texture.

18. Serotonin

19. Your circadian rhythm

20. Most experts recommend trying to get up at the same time of morning.

21. Falls

22. Late teens and early 20s. Boredom is the opposite of anxiety. Anxiety arises when one has low levels of skills and high levels of challenge.

23. Primary (or essential) hypertension

24. Mondays between 8 a.m. and 9 a.m.

25. The pacemaker known as the sinoatrial node.

26. Yes, through stress-relieving techniques, a heart-healthy diet, and exercise.

27. Malignant tumor

28. Metastasize

29. Quackery

30. Wash your hands often.

How Did You Do?

26 or more correct	You are Exceptional!!!
21 to 25 correct	You can be Proud!!!
16 to 20 correct	You should Try Harder!!!
15 or less correct	You are Not Alone!!!

Glossary

A

adenosine triphosphate (ATP) The high-energy substance found in cells from which the body gets its energy.

aerobic exercise Physical activities such as brisk walking, running, cycling, swimming, rowing, and aerobic dancing that rely heavily on oxygen for energy production.

aerobic metabolism Processes in which energy (ATP) is supplied when oxygen is utilized while a person is working.

agonist The muscle identified as the prime mover of an action.

anaerobic exercise "Without oxygen" present; short-term output of energy for muscular contraction when the oxygen supply is insufficient.

android obesity Male pattern of fat deposition in the abdominal region. Associated with cardiovascular disease and other diseases.

antagonist A muscle that causes movement at a joint in a direction opposite to that of its agonist.

arteriosclerosis An arterial disease characterized by the hardening and thickening of vessel walls.

atherosclerosis A form of arteriosclerosis in which fatty substances deposit in the inner walls of the arteries.

B

ballistic Fast, bouncy movement.

basal metabolic rate The energy required to sustain life while in a fasted and rested state.

blood pressure The force that blood exerts against the walls of the blood vessels and that makes the blood flow through the circulatory system.

blood sugar The concentrations of sugar (called glucose) in the blood.

body composition The relative amounts of muscle, bone, water, and fat in the body. Body composition is usually divided into fat and fat-free mass.

C

calorie A unit of measure for the rate of heat or energy production in the body.

carbohydrates Foodstuffs primarily used for vigorous muscular activity. Found in the body as glucose and glycogen.

cardiac output The amount of blood pumped by the heart in one minute. It is the product of heart rate and stroke volume.

cardiorespiratory endurance The capacity of your heart, blood vessels, and lungs to function optimally during sustained vigorous exercise.

cardiovascular disease A group of diseases of the heart and circulatory system.

cartilage The resilient covering of the weight-bearing surface of bones. The cartilage absorbs shock and prevents direct wear on the bones.

cellulite A label given to lumpy deposits of fat commonly appearing on the back of the legs and buttocks of some individuals.

cholesterol A fatlike substance that plays an important role as a building block for cells and hormones. It is obtained from eating foods of animal origin and also produced by the body. Elevated levels are associated with increased risk of heart disease.

circuit training Exercises performed in sequence from station to station. Usually done at a rapid pace.

contraindication A sign or symptom suggesting that a certain activity should be avoided.

cooldown An "aerobic cooldown" refers to a gradual decrease of vigorous aerobic conditioning. A "workout cooldown" refers to the stretching and relaxation phase at the end of a training session.

coronary heart disease The impairment of the coronary arteries of the heart associated with a buildup of cholesterol and fatty substances on the inner artery wall.

cross-training Selection and participation in more than one physical activity on a consistent basis.

D

dehydration The condition that results from excessive loss of water.

depression Prolonged emotional sadness that persists beyond a reasonable length of time. Often occurs with symptoms such as insomnia, headaches, exhaustion, irritability, loss of interest, impaired concentration, and feelings that life is not worth living.

diabetes mellitus A metabolic disorder in which the body is unable to regulate the level of glucose in the blood.

E

energy The capacity or ability to perform work.

exercise heart rate The heart rate during aerobic exercise that will result in cardiorespiratory benefits. Also referred to as "training heart rate."

F

fat A food substance used as an energy source. It is stored when excess fat, carbohydrate, or protein is ingested.

fiber The indigestible polysaccharides found in the leaves and stems of plants.

flexibility The range of motion of a joint or group of joints.

frequency Refers to the number of workouts needed per week to establish a training effect.

G

glucose Energy source (in the form of sugar) transported in the blood.

glycogen The form in which glucose is stored in the body (primarily in the muscles and liver).

gynoid obesity Female pattern of fat deposition in the thighs and gluteal areas that does not carry the same risk as upper body obesity.

H

heart attack Death of a part of the heart muscle caused by a lack of blood flow.

heart rate The number of times the heart beats per minute.

homeostasis The tendency of the body to maintain internal equilibrium and regulation of bodily processes.

hyperglycemia An elevation of blood sugar.

hypoglycemia Low blood sugar.

hypertension High blood pressure.

hypertrophy An increase of mass in a muscle from resistive exercise.

I

insoluble fiber Cellulose, lignin, and hemicellulose that add bulk to the contents of the intestine, accelerating the passage of food remnants through the digestive tract. Insoluble fiber may help to reduce colon cancer of the digestive tract.

intensity The level of physiological stress on the body during exercise.

isokinetic contraction A contraction in which the tension is constant throughout the range of motion.

isometric (static) contraction A contraction in which tension is developed but there is no change in the length of the muscle.

isotonic contraction A dynamic contraction in which the muscles generate force against a constant resistance.

L

lactate threshold The point during exercise when blood lactate begins to increase considerably. It is a good indicator of the highest sustainable work rate.

lactate acid The product of incomplete metabolism that can occur when insufficient oxygen is supplied to the active muscle. Believed to be a contributing factor to fatigue.

lordosis An abnormal curvature of the low back.

M

maximum heart rate The highest your heart will beat during aerobic exercise.

maximum oxygen consumption The maximal rate at which the muscles can consume oxygen in one minute.

metabolism The sum total of all physical and chemical processes occurring in the body.

mitochondria Organelles within the cells that utilize oxygen to produce ATP.

minerals Inorganic substances of the body including sodium, potassium, chloride, calcium, phosphorous, magnesium, sulfur, and at least 14 trace minerals that perform several necessary roles in the body.

monosaccharide Simple sugars such as table sugar and honey.

muscular endurance The ability to exert force (not necessarily maximal) over an extended period of time.

N

nutrients The basic substances of the body obtained by eating foods.

O

obesity An above-average amount of fat in the body. In males 25 percent or greater and in females 32 percent or greater is considered obese.

overload To exercise a muscle or group of muscles with resistance greater than normally encountered.

overtraining A condition from too much exercise characterized by a lack of energy, a decrease in performance, and bodily aches and pains.

osteoporosis The thinning and weakening of the bones that is seen predominantly in postmenopausal women.

overweight Excess weight for one's height regardless of body composition.

P

perceived exertion A subjective rating of the intensity of a particular exercise activity.

polysaccharide The joining of three or more simple sugars to form a starch.

protein A food substance that sustains basic structural properties of the cells and serves as a source for hormones and enzymes in the body.

R

recovery heart rate The gradually declining heart rate following the cessation of aerobic exercise.

repetition A repetition represents each time an exercise movement is completed.

resting heart rate The average heart rate prior to initiating any physical activity.

S

saturated fat Animal fat and fat found in dairy products and eggs that contribute to atherosclerosis.

set Group(s) of repetitions. One set might consist of 10 repetitions.

skinfold A pinch of skin and subcutaneous fat from which total body fat may be estimated.

spot reducing A myth that fat can be specifically reduced from one body area through exercise.

static stretch A stretch that is held.

strength The capacity of a muscle to exert force against resistance.

stress It is a nonspecific response of the body to pleasurable and painful demands made on it.

stretch reflex A reflexive contraction of a muscle that is being stretched.

stroke volume The amount of blood pumped by the left ventricle of the heart per beat.

T

testosterone A sex hormone appearing in much higher concentrations in males than females.

triglyceride A compound consisting of three molecules of fatty acid and glycerol. It is the main type of lipid found in the body.

U

unsaturated fat The molecules of a fat that have one or more double bonds and are thus capable of absorbing more hydrogen. These fats are usually of vegetable origin.

V

valsalva maneuver Condition occurring when a person lifts heavy weights while holding the breath. The glottis closes and intrathoracic pressure increases, hindering blood flow to the heart.

vitamins Nutrients required in microamounts that are essential to numerous bodily functions.

W

warm-up The first portion of a workout, designed to prepare the body for the vigorous exercise to follow.

The Muscle System

Muscle and Exercise Chart

This chart lists the major muscle groups and specific exercises presented in this book, as well as the opposing groups.

Deltoids
Push-up Variations
Dips
Side Lateral Raises
Chest Press
Shoulder Press

Pectorals
Chest Press
Wide-arm Push-ups
Flys

Trapezius
Power Rows

Latissimus Dorsi
Standing Rows

Biceps
Bicep Curls

Triceps
Tricep Extensions
Dips
Pike Push-ups
Chest Press

Abdominals
Crunch Variations

Obliques
Twisting Crunches
All-Around Crunches
Rope Pull Crunches

Erector Spinae
Back Extensions
Horizontal Side Bridge
Rolling Side Bridge
Bird-Dog Exercise

Gluteus Maximus
Squats
Lunges
Prone Leg Lifts
Power Exercises
Back Thigh Lifts

Rectus Femoris, Vastus Lateralis, Vastus Medialis
Squats
Lunge Variations

Biceps Femoris, Semitendinosus, Semimembranosus
Squats
Lunge Variations

Gracilis, Adductor Longus
Inner Thigh Variations
Hip Adduction
Wide Squats

Tensor Fasciae Latee, Gluteus Medius
Hip Abduction

Gastrocnemius and Soleus
Heel Raises

Examples of Opposing Muscle Groups

Biceps vs. Triceps
Deltoids vs. Latissimus Dorsi
Pectorals vs. Rhomboids and Trapezius
Quadriceps vs. Hamstrings
Abdominals vs. Spinal Extensors
Thigh Abductors vs. Thigh Adductors

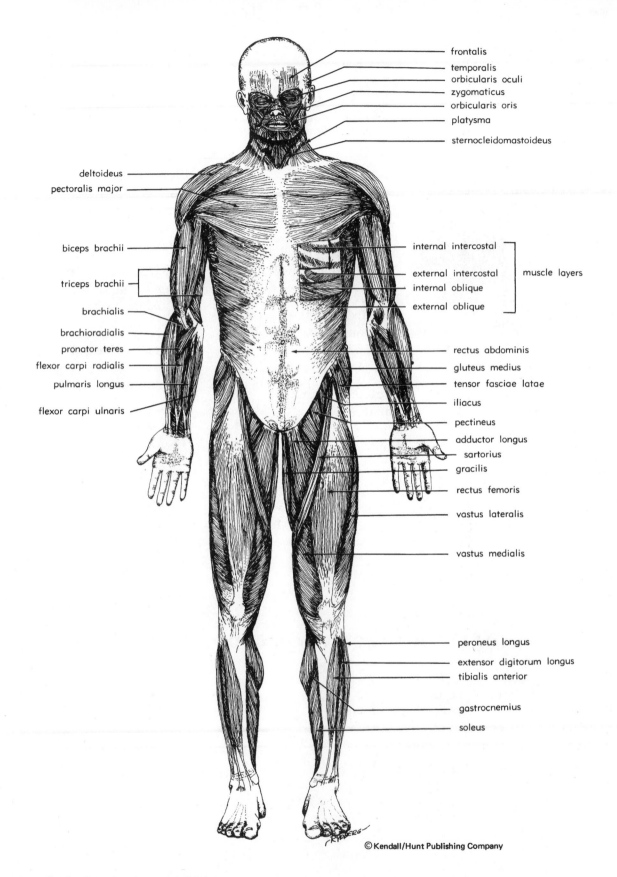

frontalis
temporalis
orbicularis oculi
zygomaticus
orbicularis oris
platysma
sternocleidomastoideus

deltoideus
pectoralis major

biceps brachii

triceps brachii

brachialis
brachioradialis
pronator teres
flexor carpi radialis
pulmaris longus
flexor carpi ulnaris

internal intercostal
external intercostal
internal oblique
external oblique

muscle layers

rectus abdominis
gluteus medius
tensor fasciae latae
iliacus
pectineus
adductor longus
sartorius
gracilis
rectus femoris
vastus lateralis
vastus medialis

peroneus longus
extensor digitorum longus
tibialis anterior
gastrocnemius
soleus

© Kendall/Hunt Publishing Company

158 Anybody's Guide to Total Fitness

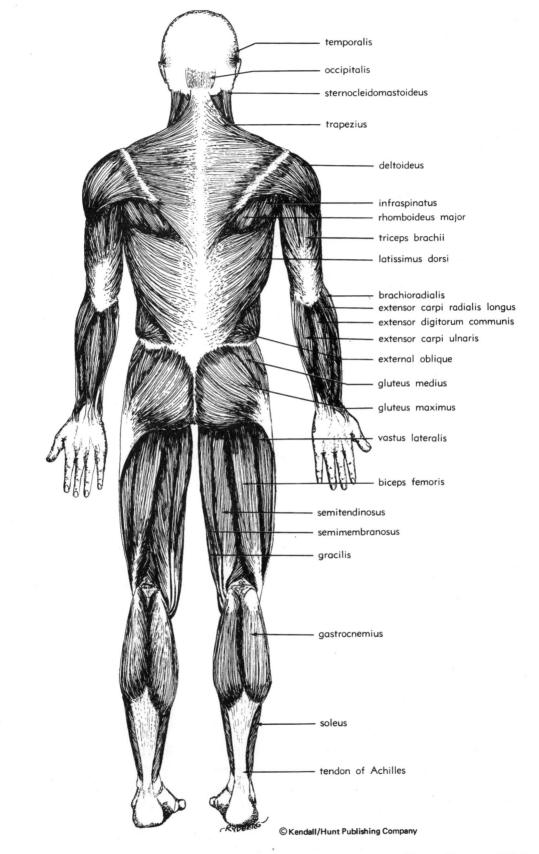

temporalis

occipitalis

sternocleidomastoideus

trapezius

deltoideus

infraspinatus
rhomboideus major
triceps brachii
latissimus dorsi

brachioradialis
extensor carpi radialis longus
extensor digitorum communis
extensor carpi ulnaris
external oblique
gluteus medius
gluteus maximus

vastus lateralis

biceps femoris

semitendinosus

semimembranosus

gracilis

gastrocnemius

soleus

tendon of Achilles

© Kendall/Hunt Publishing Company

ACSM Position Stand on Quantity and Quality of Exercise

The following is an abbreviated summary of the 1998 position stand by the American College of Sports Medicine for the recommended quantity and quality of exercise for developing and maintaining cardiorespiratory and muscular fitness, and flexibility in healthy adults.

Cardiorespiratory Fitness and Body Composition

Frequency	3 to 5 days per week
Intensity	55/65% to 90% of maximum heart rate 40/50% to 85% of maximum oxygen uptake Note: The lower intensity levels (55-64% of maximum heart rate and 40 to 49% of maximum oxygen uptake are applicable for persons with low fitness levels).
Duration	20 to 60 minutes continuous or a minimum of 10-minute bouts of accumulated exercise throughout the day
Mode	Activities that use the major muscle groups of the body in a rhythmic and continuous fashion.

Muscular Strength and Endurance and Body Composition

Frequency	2 to 3 times per week
Sets	1 set per exercise
Exercises	8 to 10 exercises for the major muscle groups of the body
Repetitions	8 to 12 repetitions for each exercise Note: For individuals approximately 50 to 60 yrs. of age and older, 10 to 15 repetitions per exercise is recommended.

Flexibility

Frequency	2 to 3 days per week
Exercises	For the major muscle groups of the body
Type	Dynamic and static stretches should be appropriately used.

Adapted from ACSM Position Stand on the Recommended Quantity and Quality of Exercise for Developing and Maintaining Cardiorespiratory and Muscular Fitness in Adults. *Medicine and Science in Sports and Exercise*, 30 (1998) 975–991.

INDEX